N

I

DATE DUE

BRODART.   Cat. No. 23-221

Nursing Process
In Clinical Practice

Springhouse Corporation
Springhouse, Pennsylvania

STAFF

Executive Director, Editorial
Stanley Loeb

Editorial Director
Matthew Cahill

Clinical Director
Barbara F. McVan, RN

Art Director
John Hubbard

Senior Editor
Michael Shaw

Clinical Editor
Joan E. Mason, RN, EdM

Editors
Jody A. Charnow, Rafaela Ellis, Traci A. Ginnona, Kathy E. Goldberg, Catherine E. Harold, Joseph E. McKendrick, Sandra Salmans, Jean Wallace

Copy Editors
Cynthia C. Breuninger (supervisor), Doris Weinstock, Priscilla DeWitt, Nancy Papsin, Christina Ponczek

Designers
Stephanie Peters (associate art director), Lorraine Carbo (book designer), Steve Karchin (cover illustrator)

Typography
David Kosten (director), Diane Paluba (manager), Elizabeth Bergman, Joyce Rossi Biletz, Phyllis Marron, Robin Mayer, Valerie Rosenberger

Manufacturing
Deborah Meiris (manager), Anna Brindisi, T.A. Landis

Production Coordination
Patricia McCloskey

Editorial Assistants
Maree DeRosa, Beverly Lane, Mary Madden

Special thanks to the George Washington University Hospital and Kaufman Advertising for use of the photograph of the nurse and patient that appears on the front cover.

NPCP-010193   ISBN 0-87434-531-6

Library of Congress
Cataloging-in-Publication Data

Nursing process in clinical practice.
    p.   cm.
    Includes bibliographical references and index.
    1. Nursing.   I. Springhouse Corporation.
    [DNLM: 1. Clinical Nursing Research. 2. Nursing Process. WY 100 N9775]
RT41.N888   1992
610.73 — dc20
DNLM/DLC   92-49070
ISBN 0-87434-531-6   CIP

CONTENTS

CONTRIBUTORS

Ruth A. Brobst, RN,C, is staff development instructor at Phoenixville (Pa.) Hospital. She is a member of the Eastern Pennsylvania Nursing Diagnosis Association.

Arlene M. Clarke Coughlin, RN, MSN, is on the nursing faculty of the Holy Name Hospital School of Nursing in Teaneck, N.J. She is a member of the American Nurses' Association, the American Association of Critical-Care Nurses, and the Urological Nurses Association.

Diane Cunningham, RN, MS, FHCE, is director of nursing education at the University of Utah Hospital in Salt Lake City. She is a member of the American Society for Health Care Education and Training and the National Nursing Staff Development Organization.

Joyce Martin Feldman, RN, MSN, is director of nursing at Overlook Hospital in Summit, N.J. She is a member of the American Association of Legal Nurse Consultants.

Robert G. Hess, Jr., RN, MSN, CCRN, CNAA, is a doctoral candidate at the University of Pennsylvania in Philadelphia, a staff nurse in the cardiovascular unit at Our Lady of Lourdes Medical Center in Camden, N.J., and a member of the adjunct faculty at Seton Hall University in South Orange, N.J. He is a member of the New Jersey State Nurses' Association, the American Nurses' Association, the American Association of Critical-Care Nurses, the Society of Critical Care Medicine, the American Organization of Nurse Executives, and the International Society of University Nurses.

Joan E. Mason, RN, EdM, is clinical editor for Springhouse Corporation in Springhouse, Pa. She is a member of the Pennsylvania Nurses' Association and the Eastern Pennsylvania Nursing Diagnosis Association.

Lois A. Fenner McBride, RN, MS, JD, is an associate with the law firm of Wright, Constable, and Skeen in Baltimore. She is treasurer of the American Association of Nurse Attorneys and a member of the American Nurses' Association, the Maryland Nurses' Association, the Maryland Trial Lawyers Association, and the American Bar Association.

Renee Perkins, RN, is resource preceptor in the resource nursing department at the University of Utah Hospital in Salt Lake City.

Carol A. Romano, RN, MS, FAAN, is director of nursing information systems and quality assurance at the Clinical Center of the National Institutes of Health in Bethesda, Md. She is a fellow of the American Academy of Nursing and a member of the American Nurses' Association's Council on Computer Applications in Nursing, the National League for Nursing Informatics Council, the American Association of Medical Informatics, and the Computer-based Patient Record Institute.

Judith J. Warren, RN, PhD, is assistant director of nursing research at University Hospital of the University of Nebraska Medical Center. She is also an associate professor at the College of Nursing of the University of Nebraska at Omaha. She is a member of the American Nurses' Association's Congress on Nursing Practice, the North American Nursing Diagnosis Association, and the American Heart Association's Council on Cardiovascular Nursing.

Wendy Wright, RN, BSN, CCRN, is charge nurse on the telemetry floor at St. Luke's Lutheran Hospital in San Antonio, Texas. She is a member of the American Association of Critical-Care Nurses, the American Nurses' Association, and the Texas Nurses' Association.

PREFACE

The nursing process fosters a systematic approach to problem solving that can benefit many areas of your professional life. For instance, the nursing process will help you apply knowledge and skills in a goal-oriented manner and thereby improve your clinical practice. It will also enhance your professional confidence and improve communication with your patients and colleagues. What's more, it will help you document care more precisely and ensure that your actions are in keeping with national standards and legal guidelines.

As the nursing profession advances, your familiarity with the nursing process will prepare you to keep pace with innovation. Indeed, this familiarity is necessary if you want to fully grasp nursing trends. That's because nursing process concepts, such as nursing diagnosis and standardized patient outcome criteria, are exerting an important influence on the development of nursing documentation systems, practice standards, nursing data bases, and computerized information systems.

In many textbooks and references, the nursing process is presented in a way that fails to stimulate the reader and often seems so removed from clinical practice as to be of limited use. However, with the publication of *Nursing Process in Clinical Practice,* you now have a book that explains the nursing process in a concise, practical, and stimulating way. Each chapter is filled with tips and tools that you can use in everyday practice. In addition, you'll find that the book's contributors — all leaders in clinical practice, education, or research — never lose sight of your most important mission: to provide the best possible patient care.

Nursing Process in Clinical Practice contains two parts, with the first covering each step of the nursing process in detail and the second covering advanced topics. Part 1 includes the first six chapters.

Chapter 1 presents an overview of the nursing process. Chapter 2, *Assessment,* discusses the purpose and content of the nursing health history and provides guidelines for developing interviewing and physical examination skills. It focuses on improving communication with the patient and overcoming barriers that interfere with the establishment of a therapeutic relationship. You'll also find numerous assessment tools as well as examples of documentation formats used to record assessment findings.

Chapter 3, *Nursing diagnosis,* explains the concepts underlying nursing diagnoses and stresses accurate use of terminology. The chapter features nine patient-focused case studies; each one shows you how to determine an appropriate nursing diagnosis.

In Chapter 4, *Planning,* you'll learn about developing the plan of care. Specifically, you'll find information on identifying expected outcomes, developing nursing interventions, soliciting patient input, and establishing priorities for care when time is limited. You'll also learn about alternative documentation formats, such as patient care protocols and critical paths.

Chapter 5, *Implementation,* describes how to put your plan of care into action. As part of this discussion, you'll learn ways to increase your professional effectiveness. Topics include acting assertively, handling professional conflicts, and strategies for collaborating with members of the health care team. This chapter also explains how to document your interventions and the patient's response to them.

Chapter 6, *Evaluation,* describes how to judge the effectiveness of nursing care and gauge the patient's progress toward meeting expected outcomes. You'll find instructions for formulating the evaluation statement, a documentation technique crucial to substantiating the rationale for nursing care.

Part 2 includes Chapters 7, 8, and 9 and covers advanced topics in the nursing process. Chapter 7 discusses discharge planning using a nursing process framework. With hospital stays growing shorter, you need a systematic approach to ensure continuity of care. Here you'll learn how to assess a patient's discharge needs, how to develop and implement a discharge plan, and how to evaluate the result of your efforts.

In Chapter 8, you'll find a discussion of important standards of practice issued by the American Nurses' Association and the Joint Commission on Accreditation of Healthcare Organizations. You'll learn about the relationship between these standards and your potential liability in a malpractice or negligence suit. This chapter also covers the legal significance of nursing documentation.

Chapter 9 discusses how computers can facilitate the nursing process. You'll find guidelines for adapting to a new computer system. You'll also learn about exciting developments in computer applications and research in nursing — developments that will have a tremendous impact on the profession's future.

At the end of Chapters 2 through 9, you'll discover key points summarized as well as a self-test that will help you evaluate your understanding of the information. Following Chapter 9, you'll find the appendices and index. The first appendix identifies all nursing diagnoses approved by the North American Nursing Diagnosis Association, including the diagnoses approved at the 10th conference in 1992. For each diagnosis, this chart gives a definition and lists the most important associated assessment findings. In the second appendix, you'll find answers with rationales for each of the self-tests.

Nurses today are entering a new era of professional responsibility. As a result, they're beginning to view themselves as autonomous professionals who can exert influence within the health care industry. Although still in the early stages of development, nursing diagnoses provide a language for describing nursing's distinctive contribution to health care.

However, if recent advances are to prove meaningful, nursing process concepts and nursing diagnoses must become familiar to all nurses and must be used when providing patient care. *Nursing Process in Clinical Practice* fulfills a crucial need by showing how to apply these concepts to clinical practice. I recommend this book for every practicing nurse and nursing student.

Judith J. Warren, RN, PhD
Associate Professor, College of Nursing
University of Nebraska at Omaha
Assistant Director of Nursing Research, University Hospital
University of Nebraska Medical Center

PART 1

UNDERSTANDING THE NURSING PROCESS

INTRODUCTION

The nursing process is a systematic approach to identifying a patient's problems and to taking nursing actions to provide solutions. Based on scientific principles, the nursing process provides a structure for accomplishing the goal of improving or maintaining the patient's well-being. (See *Fostering a problem-solving outlook.*)

You'll use the nursing process to:
• identify actual patient problems you can treat
• identify potential patient problems you can help to prevent
• develop a plan to address the patient's problems and potential problems
• determine what kind of assistance the patient requires and who can best provide it
• select goals for the patient and determine whether they've been achieved.

FROM ASSESSMENT TO EVALUATION

The nursing process consists of a series of phases or steps. Following these steps helps to identify and treat a patient's problems in an orderly and systematic way. Keep in mind, however, that these steps are dynamic and flexible—they often overlap.

The first step of the nursing process, *assessment,* includes making general observations about the patient, taking a health history, and performing a physical examination. This step is critical because the quality of assessment data will determine the success of subsequent nursing process steps.

The second step of the nursing process, *nursing diagnosis,* involves analyzing assessment findings to formulate a list of statements identifying the patient's actual or potential health problems. Each nursing diagnosis includes a diagnostic label (the problem) and a related etiology (its cause). For instance, a typical diagnostic label could be "impaired skin integrity." Its etiology could be expressed as "related to immobility." Put together, the statement would read "impaired skin integrity related to immobility."

Fostering a problem-solving outlook

The nursing process fosters a scientific approach to solving problems encountered in clinical practice. The skills employed in using it are closely related to the skills used by other professionals to identify and solve problems. The chart below shows how steps of the nursing process compare with a typical problem-solving method.

NURSING PROCESS	PROBLEM-SOLVING METHOD
Assessment • Collect and analyze subjective and objective data about the patient's health problem.	• Recognize that a problem exists. • Learn about the problem by obtaining information.
Diagnosis • State the patient's actual or potential health problems.	• State the nature of the problem.
Planning • Identify expected outcomes. • Write a plan of care that includes the nursing interventions designed to achieve expected outcomes.	• Establish goals and a time frame for achieving them. • Think of and select ways to achieve goals and solve the problem.
Implementation • Put the plan of care into action. • Document the actions taken and their results.	• Take steps to solve the problem.
Evaluation • Examine the results achieved and compare them with expected outcomes. • Review and revise the plan of care as needed.	• Decide if the actions taken have effectively solved the problem. • Revise strategies for problem solving as needed.

The third step, *planning,* involves developing a plan of care to improve or maintain the patient's health, based on the nursing diagnoses identified. Whenever possible, you'll encourage the patient to become involved in planning. Specific planning tasks include setting priorities for nursing diagnoses, identifying expected outcomes, selecting appropriate nursing interventions, and determining the time frame for achieving outcomes. During this step, you'll write the patient's plan of care.

During the next step, *implementation,* you carry out or delegate interventions outlined in the plan of care. When coordinating patient care, you may need to seek help from other caregivers, the patient, or the patient's family. You'll document nursing actions and the patient's responses to them in progress notes and flow sheets. This activity confirms that the plan of care was executed. As you carry out this step, you may identify new problems.

During *evaluation,* you analyze the results of your care, determining the extent to which expected outcomes have been achieved. To document this step, you write evaluation statements that indicate the patient's progress in meeting expected outcomes. You may need to revise the plan of care based on your findings.

Over the past few years, the steps of the nursing process have been increasingly integrated into clinical practice. For example, the American Nurses' Association's revised *Standards of Clinical Nursing Practice* states that "the nursing process encompasses all significant actions taken by nurses in providing care to all clients, and forms the foundation of clinical decision making." In addition, the Joint Commission on Accreditation of Healthcare Organizations (JCAHO) has incorporated the concept of nursing diagnosis into its revised nursing care standards. The JCAHO now requires that each patient's care be based on "nursing diagnoses and/or patient care needs and patient care standards." (See *Taking a closer look at the nursing process.*)

WHY USE THE NURSING PROCESS?
The nursing process is a powerful tool for improving clinical practice. It can, for instance, help you develop an innovative outlook on patient care, foster cooperation with patients and colleagues, and improve documentation. What's more, the nursing process can strengthen your professional identity.

Developing an open and innovative outlook
Although firmly rooted in scientific principles, the nursing process offers an open approach to addressing patient problems. It provides a structure for problem solving without limiting you to a specific theoretical framework.

The nursing process encourages you to become more innovative in providing care. For example, suppose that while working in a long-term care facility, you encounter an elderly patient whose treatment regimen relies too heavily on the use

Taking a closer look at the nursing process

The chart below depicts the steps of the nursing process as well as the discrete aspects of each step. As you read this chart, keep in mind the cyclical nature of the nursing process. The sequence of steps repeats itself until the patient's nursing needs have been addressed.

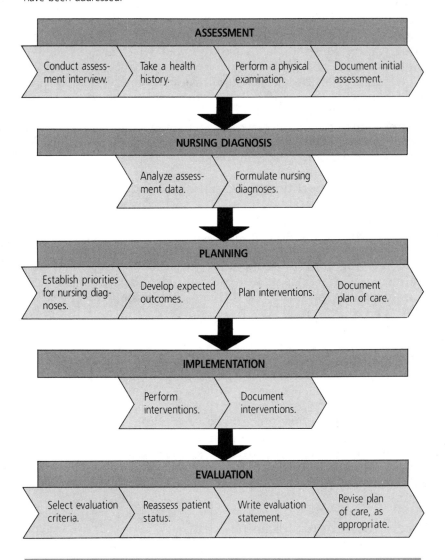

ASSESSMENT

Conduct assessment interview.

Take a health history.

Perform a physical examination.

Document initial assessment.

NURSING DIAGNOSIS

Analyze assessment data.

Formulate nursing diagnoses.

PLANNING

Establish priorities for nursing diagnoses.

Develop expected outcomes.

Plan interventions.

Document plan of care.

IMPLEMENTATION

Perform interventions.

Document interventions.

EVALUATION

Select evaluation criteria.

Reassess patient status.

Write evaluation statement.

Revise plan of care, as appropriate.

of psychotropic drugs to help her cope with mild depression. You suspect that the patient's emotional state is related more to loneliness and stress than to biochemical factors. To more accurately reflect this patient's nursing care needs, you can use the nursing process to formulate a plan of care that places greater emphasis on psychosocial interventions.

Taking the time to develop a nursing diagnosis gives you the advantage of formulating a hypothesis before planning your interventions. It offers a bridge between the need for clear thinking and the need for effective action. For example, suppose you're caring for a diabetic patient who initially seems stubborn and doesn't comply with his therapeutic regimen. However, after taking a thorough history, you find that the patient has never learned the relationship between blood glucose control and diet, medication, and exercise. You would then write a nursing diagnosis that accurately describes the patient's knowledge deficit and specify nursing interventions to address the patient's learning needs.

Fostering cooperation with patients and colleagues
When using the nursing process, the patient's individual health care needs, not his disease, become the focus of care. This emphasis promotes the patient's participation and encourages his independence and compliance—factors important to a positive outcome. You may also find that you're better able to communicate with colleagues. After all, identifying a patient's nursing needs provides a common goal among nurses who care for the patient. What's more, documenting your findings helps to ensure continuity of care.

Improving documentation
Familiarity with the nursing process will also improve your documentation of care. Using a nursing-oriented approach to documentation helps to ensure that your contribution to the patient's well-being is recognized. Including precise patient outcome statements in your plan of care helps to foster accountability for nursing activities, thereby promoting improved quality of care. For nurses, accepting greater accountability is part and parcel of gaining professional recognition.

Strengthening professional identity
Since the time of Florence Nightingale, nurses have struggled with such questions as "What is nursing?" and "Is nursing

truly a profession?" Although the image of a nurse as a helper and caregiver has become ingrained in the public mind, nurses have had difficulty asserting their identity as autonomous professionals who apply knowledge and judgment when carrying out medical orders and who must make numerous independent clinical decisions.

The nursing process developed partly in response to the need of nurses to define their role within the health care system. Today, the nursing process provides a model for promoting the professional status of nurses. It shows how to apply knowledge and skills in an organized, goal-oriented manner. It also clearly defines the problems nurses treat independently. What's more, it helps to identify nursing's contribution to collaborative practice.

In addition, the development of nursing diagnoses has contributed to establishing nursing as a distinct profession with its own body of knowledge. Becoming familiar with nursing diagnosis terminology will clarify what nurses do and how their practice differs from that of doctors and other health care professionals.

ASSESSMENT

Performing a patient assessment is your first task when carrying out the nursing process. It serves as your opportunity to lay the foundation necessary for achieving excellence in clinical practice. All subsequent steps of the nursing process as well as the quality of your patient care depend on the strength of your nursing assessment.

This chapter provides guidelines for a broad range of assessment activities: observing the patient, interviewing him, gathering health history data, assessing physiologic systems, interviewing family members, and performing the physical examination.

The quality of your assessment depends largely on your ability to communicate effectively with the patient. Your assessment interview is not intended to be a question and answer session, but a meaningful dialogue. To encourage the patient to open up to you, you'll have to communicate empathy, maintain objectivity, and eliminate any cultural biases. You'll find instructions for sharpening communication skills in various patient contact situations.

You will also find detailed information on how to document assessment findings, including examples of the various documentation formats currently in use. Your assessment documentation should form a complete picture of the patient. Accurately recorded assessment information will help you proceed smoothly through the remaining steps of the nursing process — especially when it's time to formulate nursing diagnoses and create an effective plan of care.

CLASSIFYING ASSESSMENT DATA

During your assessment, you'll need to distinguish between two types of data — subjective and objective. Subjective information represents the patient's perception of his problem, such as a complaint of chest pain. Objective information is data you can observe or measure and can verify. A patient's blood pressure reading is objective information. During your assessment, you'll gather both types of information from primary and secondary sources.

Subjective data

Subjective data usually include the patient's chief complaint or concern, current health status, health history, family history, psychosocial history, activities of daily living, and review of body systems.

The patient's history, embodying his perception of his problems, is your most important source of assessment information. But it's also subjective, so you must interpret it carefully. Suppose, for instance, that a patient complains of "frequent stomach pain." To find out what he considers "frequent," ask if the pain occurs once a week, once a day, twice a day, or all day. To find out what he means by "stomach," have him point to the specific area affected. This will also tell you if the pain is localized or generalized. To find out how he defines "pain," have him describe the sensation. Is it stabbing or dull, twisting or nagging? How does he rate its severity on a scale of 1 to 10?

When documenting subjective information, be sure to record it as such. Whenever possible, write the patient's own words in quotation marks. And introduce patient statements with a phrase such as "Patient states." For instance, you would document the previous example like this:

"Patient states that he has 'frequent stomach pain.' He describes pain as 'dull and nagging.' Patient rates pain as a 4 on a scale of 1 to 10. The pain occurs after eating, is relieved by antacids, and is located in the left lower quadrant."

If the patient uses unfamiliar words or phrases, such as slang words, ask him to define them. For clarity, record both the phrase and the patient's definition of it.

To fully explore a patient's complaint, use the "PQRST" memory device as a guide. By using a standard format of questions about the nature of his symptoms, you'll prompt the patient to describe his symptoms in greater detail. (See *Clarifying subjective information*, page 10.)

Objective data

Objective information, unlike subjective data, doesn't require interpretation. If another practitioner were to make the same observations under the same circumstances, she would obtain the same information. Be specific and avoid using subjective

Clarifying subjective information

To fully explore a patient's complaint, use the PQRST memory device as a guide. When you ask the questions listed here, you'll prompt the patient to describe his symptoms in greater detail. Only when you have such clarifying detail can you properly interpret this subjective information.

P	**PROVOCATIVE OR PALLIATIVE** • What were you doing when you first experienced or noticed the symptom? What seems to trigger it: stress? position? certain activities? arguments? • What makes the symptom worse? • What relieves the symptom: changing diet? changing position? taking medication? being active?
Q	**QUALITY OR QUANTITY** • How would you describe the symptom — how it feels, looks, or sounds? • How much are you experiencing now? Is it so much that it prevents you from performing any activities? Is it more or less than you experienced at any other time?
R	**REGION OR RADIATION** • Where does the symptom occur? • Does it spread? In the case of pain, does it travel down your back or arms, up your neck, or down your legs?
S	**SEVERITY SCALE** • How would you rate the symptom at its worst on a scale of 1 to 10, with 10 being the most severe? Does it force you to lie down, sit down, or slow down? • Does the symptom seem to be getting better, getting worse, or staying about the same?
T	**TIMING** • On what date did the symptom first occur? What time did it begin? • How did the symptom start: suddenly? gradually? • How often do you experience the symptom: hourly? daily? weekly? monthly? • When do you usually experience it: during the day? at night? in the early morning? Does it awaken you? Does it occur before, during, or after meals? Does it occur seasonally? • How long does an episode of the symptom last?

terms, such as "large," "small," or "moderate," when documenting objective information. Whenever possible, use measurements to record data clearly. Specify color, size, and location when appropriate. For instance, "small amount of abdominal wound drainage" could be more clearly described as "about ½ teaspoon of serosanguineous abdominal wound drainage."

Avoid interpreting the data and reflecting your opinion. For example, don't write that the "patient is in shock." Instead, document the findings: "pale skin, pulse rate of 140, blood pressure of 90/60 mm Hg."

TAKING A NURSING HEALTH HISTORY

The major source of information about a patient's health status, the nursing health history may include physiologic, psychological, cultural, and psychosocial data. It provides a guide to the physical examination that follows.

The nursing health history is distinguished by its holistic focus on the human response to illness. Whereas a medical history is designed to guide diagnosis and treatment of illness, your purpose in obtaining a health history includes planning health care, assessing the impact of illness on the patient and family, evaluating patient health education needs, and initiating discharge planning.

Several different formats exist for conducting a nursing health history. Each format provides a logical sequence for the interview and an organized record of the patient's responses. The major distinction is that some formats reflect the medical model, whereas others are more deeply rooted in nursing practice. Using a nursing assessment framework may prove especially useful when seeking to develop nursing diagnoses. Although there is debate about which framework works best, all nursing assessment models take into account psychological and social aspects of the patient's experience.

The functional health patterns developed by Marjory Gordon in 1982 provide one example of a nursing approach to collecting health history data. Gordon groups health history data into 11 categories called patterns. This system allows for easy organization of basic nursing information obtained during the initial assessment. Flexible and adaptable, these functional health patterns can be used for patients in various states of health and illness, in any age-group, and in any clinical specialty. (See *Using Gordon's functional health patterns to structure your assessment*, pages 12 to 15.)

(Text continues on page 15.)

Using Gordon's functional health patterns to structure your assessment

Nursing theorist Marjory Gordon has identified 11 functional health patterns that you can use to structure your nursing assessment data base. Gordon's system allows for easy organization of assessment information.

When using Gordon's approach, you will evaluate the patient's functioning in 11 areas: health perception and health management, nutrition and metabolism, elimination, activity and exercise, sleep and rest, cognition and perception, self-perception and self-concept, roles and relationships, sexuality and reproduction, coping and stress tolerance, and values and beliefs. Your evaluation will be based on the patient interview and your own observations.

The patient interview
The list below provides an example of how you might use Gordon's functional health patterns to organize your questions during a patient interview.

Health perception and health management pattern
• How is your general health?
• Have you had any illnesses in the past year? Have you been absent from work?
• What do you do to keep healthy? Do you believe your actions make a difference to your health? (Discuss family folk remedies, if appropriate.)
• Do you use cigarettes, alcohol, or drugs?
• Do you conduct regular breast self-examinations (female patient)?
• Have you had any recent accidents (home, work, driving)?
• Have you found it easy to follow doctors' or nurses' instructions?
• What do you think caused your current illness? What actions did you take when you first perceived the symptoms? What were the results of these actions?
• What things are most important to you during your stay at this facility? How can the nursing staff be most helpful to you?

Nutritional and metabolic pattern
• Describe your typical daily food intake. Do you take any supplements, such as vitamins? What types of snacks do you eat?
• Describe your typical daily fluid intake.
• What has been your most recent weight loss or gain?
• How is your appetite?
• Do you experience any discomfort in eating or swallowing?
• Do you have any diet restrictions?
• Do you heal well or poorly?
• Do you have any skin problems, such as lesions or dryness?
• Do you have any dental problems?

Using Gordon's functional health patterns to structure your assessment — continued

Elimination pattern
• Describe your bowel elimination pattern, including frequency, character of stools, discomfort, problem in control, and use of laxatives.
• Describe your urinary elimination pattern, including frequency and problem in control.
• Do you experience any excess perspiration or odor problems?

Activity and exercise pattern
• Do you have sufficient energy for daily activities?
• Describe your exercise habits. What types of exercises do you engage in?
• What are your spare time or leisure activities?
• Consider each of the activities listed below. Can you complete the activity independently? Can you complete the activity with partial assistance? Do you require any special equipment or device to perform the activity?
  — Feeding
  — Grooming
  — Bathing
  — Toileting
  — Cooking
  — Home maintenance
  — Dressing
  — Shopping

Sleep and rest pattern
• In general, do you feel rested and ready for daily activities after sleep?
• Do you have any sleep onset problems? Do you use any aids to help you sleep? What kinds of dreams or nightmares do you have? Are you subject to early awakenings?
• Do you regularly set aside time for rest and relaxation? What types of activities do you find relaxing?

Cognitive and perceptual pattern
• Do you have any hearing difficulties? Do you use a hearing aid?
• How is your vision? Do you wear glasses? When were your eyes last checked?
• If you wear glasses or contact lenses, when was your prescription last changed?
• Have you experienced any change in your ability to remember?
• Do you have any difficulty making big decisions?
• What is the easiest way for you to learn things? Do you experience any difficulty when trying to learn something new?
• If you experience any discomfort or pain, how do you manage it?

(continued)

Using Gordon's functional health patterns to structure your assessment – *continued*

Self-perception and self-concept pattern
• How would you describe yourself? How do you feel about yourself most of the time?
• Is there anything about yourself or your appearance you would like to change?
• Has your illness affected the way you feel about yourself or your body?
• Do you frequently feel angry, annoyed, fearful, anxious, depressed, or out of control? What helps alleviate these feelings?
• Do you ever lose hope?

Role and relationship pattern
• Do you live alone or with others?
• Do you have a close family? (Consider asking the patient to make a diagram of his family structure.)
• Have you had difficulty handling problems with your nuclear or extended family?
• Do family members or others depend on you? How are they managing while you are ill?
• What feelings have family members and friends expressed about your illness or hospitalization?

Sexuality and reproductive pattern
• Are your sexual relationships satisfying? Have any changes or problems taken place with these relationships? (Make sure questions are appropriate to patient's age and situation.)
• Do you use contraceptives? Have you had any problems with this use?
• When was your last menstrual period? Are you having any menstrual problems? Do you have any children? Are you currently pregnant? (Female patient)

Coping and stress tolerance pattern
• Have you experienced any big changes or crises in your life in the last 2 years?
• Who do you turn to for help during a personal crisis? Is anyone available to help you now?
• Do you feel tense much of the time? What helps to alleviate tension?
• Do you use medications, drugs, or alcohol to enhance your ability to cope?
• How do you handle major problems in your life? Do you handle problems successfully most of the time?

Value and belief pattern
• Do you generally get what you want from life? Do you have plans for the future?
• Is religion important in your life? If so, does it help when difficulties arise?
• Will your hospitalization interfere with your religious practices?

Using Gordon's functional health patterns to structure your assessment — *continued*

Observations and physical examination findings
The list below provides an example of how you might use Gordon's functional health patterns to organize observations made during the assessment and physical examination.

Nutritional and metabolic pattern
• Weight
• Height
• Temperature
• Need for parenteral nutrition
• Skin (bony prominences, lesions)
• Oral mucous membranes (color, moistness, lesions)
• Teeth (dentures, cavities, missing)

Activity and exercise pattern
• Gait
• Posture
• Hand grip
• Coordination
• Range of motion
• Muscle firmness
• Use of prostheses
• Use of assistive equipment
• Pulse rate, rhythm
• Respiratory rate, depth, rhythm
• Breath sounds
• Blood pressure

Cognitive and perceptual pattern
• Grasp of ideas, questions
• Language spoken
• Hearing
• Vision
• Orientation
• Vocabulary
• Attention span

Self-perception and self-concept pattern
• Body posture
• Voice and speech pattern
• Eye contact
• Nervous or relaxed

Role and relationship pattern
• Interactions with family members, friends, others
• Assertive or passive

Observing the patient
You can obtain important information by carefully observing the patient. Begin as soon as you meet him. You may, for example, observe the patient while taking him to his room. Continue to make general observations during the interview and physical examination as well as throughout the patient's hospitalization. By looking critically at the patient, you can collect valuable information about his emotional state, comfort level, and physical condition. (See *Making general observations,* page 16.)

Making general observations

Your general observations of the patient's appearance, cognitive functions, communication ability, and mobility are an important part of your initial assessment. The following are the specific characteristics to look for and to document.

Appearance

Age
• Appears to be stated age
• Appears older or younger than stated age

Physical condition
• Physically fit, strong, and appropriate weight for height
• Out of shape, weak, and either underweight or overweight
• Apparent limitations, such as an amputation or paralysis
• Obvious scars or rash

Dress
• Dressed appropriately or inappropriately for season
• Clean and well-kept clothes
• Soiled or torn clothes that smell of alcohol, urine, or feces

Personal hygiene
• Clean and well groomed
• Unkempt; dirty skin, hair, and nails; unshaved
• Body odor or unusual breath odor

Skin color
• Pale, ruddy, cyanotic, jaundiced, or tanned

Cognitive functions

Awareness
• Oriented; aware of surroundings
• Disoriented; unaware of person, place, or time

Mood
• Responds appropriately; talkative
• Answers in one-word responses; offers information only in response to direct questions
• Hesitant to answer questions; looks to family member before answering
• Angry; states "Leave me alone" (or similar response); speaks loudly and abruptly to family members
• Maintains, or avoids, eye contact

Thought processes
• Maintains a conversation; makes relevant statements; follows commands appropriately
• Mind seems to wander; makes irrelevant statements; follows commands inappropriately

Communication

Speech
• Speaks clearly in English or other language
• Speaks only with one-word responses; doesn't respond to verbal stimuli
• Speech seems slurred, hoarse, loud, soft, incoherent, hesitant, slow, fast, or nonsensical
• Has difficulty completing sentences because of shortness of breath or pain

Hearing
• Hears well enough to respond to questions
• Hard of hearing; wears hearing aid; must be spoken to loudly into left or right ear
• Deaf; reads lips or uses sign language

Vision
• Sees well enough to read instructions in English or other language
• Wears glasses to see or to read
• Can't read
• Blind

Mobility

Ambulation
• Walks independently; steady gait
• Uses a cane, crutches, or walker
• Unsteady, slow, hesitant, or shuffling gait; leans toward one side; can't support own weight
• Transfers from chair to bed independently
• Needs assistance (from one, two, or three people) to transfer from chair to bed

Movement
• Moves all extremities
• Has right- or left-sided weakness; paralysis
• Can't turn in bed independently
• Has jerky or spastic movements of body parts (specify)

Conducting a successful patient interview

Your interview with the patient is a vital part of the health history. Data gathered during the patient interview is essential for developing a plan of care tailored to the patient's needs.

As you prepare for the interview, consider the patient's ability and readiness to participate. For example, if he's sedated or confused, hostile or angry, or experiencing pain or dyspnea, ask only the most essential questions. You can perform a more in-depth interview later, when his condition improves. In the meantime, secondary sources can often provide much of the needed information.

The interview has three parts—the introduction, body, and closure. During the introduction, you initiate your relationship with the patient. Projecting a professional attitude from the beginning is crucial. Try to alleviate as much of the patient's discomfort and anxiety as possible. Create a quiet, private environment. Avoid interruptions by arranging for another nurse to cover your other patients during the interview. Your efforts will communicate to the patient that you're interested in and respect the confidentiality of what he tells you.

Tell the patient how long the interview will last—usually from 15 to 30 minutes for a medical-surgical patient. Explain the purpose of the history so that he understands why you'll be asking him personal questions. Finally, be calm, relaxed, and unhurried. Your actions will convey to the patient the importance of the health history interview. (See *Making the most of your interview time,* page 18.)

During the body of the interview, you obtain the required information. In most cases, you'll begin with the patient's chief complaint and move into other areas, such as medical and family histories.

During the final—or closure—phase, you wrap up the interview and summarize the points that were discussed. This gives the patient the opportunity to agree or disagree with your perceptions of his health status and concerns. This also helps you develop expected outcomes for your plan of care.

Effective interviewing techniques

Examples of effective interviewing techniques are listed below. Remember, however, that techniques that work in one situation may not be effective in another.
• *Offer general leads.* General questions give the patient an opportunity to speak freely. Such questions as "What brought you here today?" or "Are you concerned about any other

Making the most of your interview time

In today's busy and frequently understaffed health care environment, it's often difficult to conduct a thorough patient interview. Certain strategies, however, can help
you make the most of the time you have without compromising quality.

Consider asking the patient to complete a questionnaire about his past and present health status. Then you can quickly and easily document his health history by reviewing the information on the questionnaire. This method has been most successful
in short procedures units and before admission for elective procedures. Although it
saves time, this method doesn't give you an opportunity to develop a therapeutic relationship with your patient.

If you must conduct an interview but are pressed for time, the following tips will
help you obtain a health history more quickly:
• Gather preinterview data. Before the interview, fill in as much of the health history
information as you can from secondary sources, such as admission forms, transfer
summaries, and the medical history. This avoids duplication of effort and reduces interview time. If some of this information needs clarification, you can ask the patient
for a fuller explanation. For instance, you might say, "You told Dr. Smith that you
have periodic dizzy spells. Can you tell me more about those spells?"
• Seek assistance where appropriate. Check your facility's policy regarding who can
gather assessment data. You may be able to have a nursing assistant or an LPN collect routine information about such things as allergies and past hospitalizations. Remember, however, that you must review the information and verify it as necessary.
• Focus on the chief complaint. Begin the interview by asking about the patient's
chief complaint and the reason for his hospitalization. Then, if the interview is interrupted, you'll have some initial information on which to base a plan of care.
• Follow the form. Use your facility's nursing assessment documentation form as a
guide to organize information. Ask your patient only pertinent questions.
• Take only brief notes during the interview. This avoids interrupting the flow of conversation. Complete longer summations or expand on information as soon as possible after you complete the interview. You can always go back to the patient if you
need to clarify or verify information.
• Keep it short and simple. Record your findings in concise, specific phrases, and use
approved abbreviations.

things?" will prompt the patient to open up and do most of the
talking. Provide ample time for reflection and response. Comments such as "Please continue" or "What happened next?" encourage the patient to share his thoughts.

• *Restate the essence of the patient's comments.* This will help
you to interpret the patient's statement more accurately or obtain additional insight. For example:

Patient: The doctor told me to take my medication twice a day.

Nurse: I see; you take Bactrim once in the morning and once at night.

Patient: No, I take it at 8 a.m. and at noon because he said twice a day.

In this situation, restating the patient's words led to an opportunity to clarify misconceptions about his drug regimen.

• *Focus the discussion.* To help the patient identify significant health concerns, focus on important points. For example:

Nurse: What do you do for a living?

Patient: I'm a coal miner.

Nurse: Are you aware of any health hazards in coal mining?

• *Encourage the patient to express himself.* By encouraging the expression of opinions, concerns, and doubts, you affirm the patient's individual value.

• *Seek clarification of vague or confusing remarks.* This will help avoid misinterpreting the patient's needs. If necessary, admit that you don't understand what the patient is saying. Ask questions to clarify the patient's descriptions of symptoms — for example, "Was the mole as big as a dime?" If the patient makes unrealistic statements or exaggerates, pointing out reality usually encourages him to modify his statements. For example:

Patient: I never get anything to eat.

Nurse: But Mr. Johnson, when we discussed your eating habits, you told me that you had three meals a day.

Patient: I meant that I never get anything to eat that I like.

• *State observations about the patient's behavior.* Your words may increase the patient's awareness of his situation or open new areas for discussion. For example, the observation "I notice that you are rubbing your eyes a lot. Do they bother you?" may lead to a discussion of allergies, vision problems, or altered sleep patterns.

• *Use silence when appropriate.* A period of silence may help the patient organize his thoughts and consider what to say next, while allowing you an opportunity to observe. Using silence effectively may even convey empathy. Although long silences can be awkward, avoid saying something just to reduce anxiety.

• *Summarize each health history component before moving to a new topic.* This helps clarify information and ease the transition between topics. For example:

Nurse: That completes the family history section. I've noted that your father and grandfather died of heart attacks and your maternal grandmother had a stroke. Everyone else in your immediate family is alive and healthy, except for your paternal grandmother who has diabetes. Is that correct?
Patient: Yes, that's right.
Nurse: Okay, let's review your physiologic status.

Communication cautions

Poor interviewing techniques create communication problems between you and the patient. Consider the guidelines listed below.
• *Avoid asking why or how questions.* Such questions force the patient to justify feelings and thoughts. A question that begins with "why" or "how" may be perceived as a threat or a challenge; the patient may feel that he should invent an answer if he does not have one. For example:

Patient: I really feel awful this morning — I just get so incredibly depressed these days.
Nurse: Why do you think you become depressed so often?
This question asks for an insight that the patient may not have. Instead, ask for information that the patient can supply more readily — for example, "Can you tell me more about what it's like when you're depressed?"
• *Avoid probing, persistent questioning.* This style of questioning may increase patient discomfort, create defensive feelings, and make the patient feel manipulated. One or two attempts to elicit information about a particular topic are sufficient.

Nurse: Let's discuss your overall health. Can you tell me about any past illnesses?
Patient: Well, I had my appendix out, I had scarlet fever, and I was in the hospital for a mental problem.
Nurse: What mental problem?
Patient: Manic depression.
Nurse: What was that like?
Patient: Oh, I don't know. I don't like to think about it.
Nurse: What did you do in your manic phases?
Here, the nurse is asking questions that have little relevance to the patient's overall health status. Once the patient names his mental illness, no further explanations are required.
• *Don't use inappropriate language.* Avoid using technical jargon or abstract terms that are incompatible with the patient's developmental level, education, or background. The patient may

perceive this as an unwillingness to share information or an attempt to hide something.

• *Avoid giving advice.* Sharing personal experiences or opinions and giving advice imply that you know what is best for the patient; this may discourage the patient from participating in health care decisions. In many cases, a patient who asks for advice has already made a decision and wants a sounding board for ideas. For example, if a patient asks whether a surgical procedure should be performed, avoid giving advice. Instead, ask, "What would you like to do?" or "What thoughts do you have about it?"

• *Don't give false reassurance.* Glib remarks, such as "Everything will be fine," communicate a lack of sensitivity. Avoid offering false reassurance to relieve your anxiety if you can't help the patient. If a patient expresses fear or anguish about his medical diagnosis or treatment, you should simply and compassionately acknowledge his feelings.

Avoid using clichés, such as "You'll feel better in the morning" or "Where there's life there's hope." These phrases may discourage the patient from expressing genuine feelings.

• *Don't change the subject or interrupt.* Such behavior indicates a lack of empathy. Interrupting the patient's idea flow may confuse him. Wait until the patient completes a thought before clarifying a relevant point.

• *Don't give excessive approval if you agree with the patient's remarks.* Telling the patient that a response is particularly good implies that an opposing response is bad. It may set narrow limits on other patient responses by encouraging answers that will gain approval. Be careful to express approval of the patient's remarks in an appropriate manner.

• *Don't make hasty conclusions.* Doing so will only invite inadequate or inaccurate information. For example:

Patient: I've had three cans of beer a day for the last 10 years.

Nurse: I'm glad you've decided to come to us for help. It shows that you're sincerely ready to quit drinking.

In this example, the patient may be reluctant to provide additional assessment information because he fears the nurse's disapproval.

• *Avoid becoming defensive.* A patient may express anger and frustration about his treatment, the facility, or the staff. A defensive response from you implies that the patient has no right to express such feelings and may increase the patient's anger. Consider the following exchange:

Patient: The care I received in that hospital was terrible. No one ever answered my call light, and I had to wait hours for a pain pill.

Nurse: I'm sure no one meant to ignore you. Nurses get so busy, sometimes they can't do as much as they'd like.

Instead of defending the nursing profession, show empathy by saying, for example, "That must have been a difficult experience."

• *Don't ask leading questions.* By its phrasing, a leading question suggests the "right" answer, as in the question "You've never had a sexually transmitted disease, have you?"

This type of question may force the patient to supply a socially acceptable response rather than an honest one.

Overcoming communication barriers

A variety of problems may interfere with your ability to communicate with the patient. You may need to make a special effort to overcome communication barriers to conduct a successful patient interview. Below you'll find guidelines for communicating effectively with patients with hearing deficits, elderly patients, patients with serious illnesses or injuries (including those that require attachment to life-support systems), and patients from unfamiliar cultures. Keep in mind, however, that there are no set formulas for opening up lines of communication. Your efforts to overcome obstacles to a therapeutic relationship should be individualized for each patient.

Hearing-impaired and elderly patients

Hearing deficits are one of the most common barriers to successful communication, especially with elderly patients: 30% to 60% of all older people experience progressive hearing loss. The following guidelines will assist you in communicating with hearing-impaired and certain elderly patients:

• Face the patient when speaking with him.

• Speak more slowly than usual and keep your voice pitch normal. Many older or hearing-impaired patients can't discriminate words if you speak quickly or in a high-pitched voice. Do not, however, speak so slowly that you make the patient feel stupid.

• Keep your hands away from your face when you speak and enunciate each word clearly. A hearing-impaired or elderly patient may understand you better if he can read your lips.

• If the patient has a hearing aid, be sure that it is clean and has a functioning battery. If the patient can't adjust the volume, take the hearing aid out of his ear, turn the volume dial until it emits a ringing sound, and adjust it in the opposite direction until the ringing is suppressed.

• Announce yourself when you enter the room or approach the patient. Say the patient's name loud enough so he can hear you and respond, especially if he is hearing-impaired. Don't shout, and don't get his attention by walking up to him and touching his arm—you'll only startle him.

• If appropriate, make sure the patient's eyeglasses are clean and within reach. Also make sure the patient puts his eyeglasses on when you're speaking to him.

• Ask the patient to turn off his television or radio before you speak to him, or find another quieter place to talk. Note that many older patients lose the ability to tune out or interpret distracting noises.

• When you begin to talk, announce the subject—for example, "I'd like to talk with you about your medications." To a certain degree, a hearing-impaired person relies on predictability in conversation. By knowing the subject of the conversation, your patient will recognize words that might otherwise be unclear to him.

• If you must use unfamiliar words, such as medical terms, write them down. This may make sounds that are strange understandable to the patient.

• Wait quietly for an elderly patient to answer your questions. He may be slow to understand the meaning of the words, even if he has heard them clearly. Likewise, don't rush him if he's struggling to express his thoughts. Demonstrate tact and a willingness to listen. Even if you can't understand the patient, let him know that you accept his efforts to communicate and that you empathize with his frustration.

Critically ill or injured patients

A patient may have difficulty communicating with you as a result of illness, injury, or attachment to life-support systems. For example, the patient may have experienced aphasia as a result of a stroke or may be progressively losing his speech from a neuromuscular disease such as Guillain-Barré syndrome. For the ventilator patient, temporary loss of speech may be a terrifying experience, even though members of the hospital staff treat it as a routine postoperative condition. Because providing technical care to a seriously ill patient can be so demanding, overcoming communication barriers may seem secondary. However, even a seriously ill patient deserves the opportunity to contribute to his plan of care as much as possible.

If the patient is in the intensive care unit, make sure he understands where he is and what's happening to him. If he's connected to life-support equipment, be sure he understands why. For example, a patient who has had an endotracheal tube inserted during a respiratory emergency won't be able to think about communicating with you until he understands why he can't speak. Keep in mind that speaking slowly and loudly will not help you transcend the communication barrier with a ventilator patient; the patient isn't deaf or unaware.

When initiating communication with a seriously ill or injured patient, begin with yes-or-no questions so that the patient will be able to answer easily. If the patient is hooked up to life-support systems or cannot talk, determine how he wants to respond to your questions: nodding for yes and shaking his head for no, moving his eyes up for yes and down for no, or wiggling his fingers. Blinking may not be useful as a communication method — a reflex blink could be confused with an answer.

If you must repeat questions, do so quietly and calmly, using gestures and facial expressions to reinforce the message you're trying to convey. Allow extra time for the patient to respond. Resist the impulse to talk to the patient like a child. If the patient is aphasic, try not to embarrass him by correcting his speech.

Through your words and actions, demonstrate to the patient that you understand the nature of his condition. For example, you might say, "I know that you know what you want to say." In this way, you make it clear that you don't suspect him of being unintelligent and that you realize his mind is working clearly. This will help the patient's self-esteem.

Using communication aids may help a speech-impaired patient to express himself. Examples of such aids include the following:
• Paper, clipboard, and felt-tip pen. Attach the pen to the clipboard so that it can't fall out of the patient's reach.
• Magic slates. These resemble flip charts with a clear plastic sheet stapled to a waxed black surface. Any blunt instrument can be used for a pen, such as a tongue blade, a needle cap, or an applicator with the wooden end wrapped in silk tape.
• Alphabet board. If a patient's poor eyesight impairs his handwriting ability, or if he doesn't have the strength or coordination to write legibly, he may be able to communicate by

pointing to the letters of the alphabet. Try printing the alphabet on a piece of cardboard and asking him to point out letters to create words. On the back of the board, draw pictures of some common needs (bedpan, glass of water, and so on).
• Word cards. On each page of a 4" × 6" cardboard flip chart, write a common word or phrase that the patient may want to use.

Cultural barriers
Until recently, health care providers paid little attention to the health beliefs and practices of members of ethnic and minority cultures. Consequently, many cultural minority groups were reluctant to seek health care services, preferring instead to use home remedies and coming to the hospital as a last resort. Today, doctors, nurses, social workers, and other health care professionals realize that cultural beliefs and values can greatly influence health care outcomes. When nursing care is culturally relevant, patients are more likely to understand and follow through with health teaching.

Throughout your career, you will be called upon to assess, care for, and work with people of many different cultures. Keep in mind that diversity exists not just between cultures but within cultures and between generations. Performing a cultural assessment will help you work more effectively with patients of different backgrounds by heightening your awareness of and sensitivity to the health beliefs and practices of these patients. The assessment consists of questions about the patient's cultural affiliation, health care beliefs and practices, illness beliefs and customs, interpersonal relations, spiritual practices, world view, and life-style. (See *Performing a cultural assessment*, pages 26 and 27.)

Language barriers
Language differences and dialects may also interfere with your ability to communicate with the patient. Even among people who speak the same language, culturally based word connotations can create confusion. You should try to become familiar with the languages spoken by patient groups in your clinical practice setting. If necessary, enlist the help of someone, such as a friend or family member of the patient, who can serve as translator.

Socioeconomic, educational, and developmental background may all affect the patient's speech. For example, the patient may have a limited vocabulary, or jargon or slang may dom-

Performing a cultural assessment

The following questions provide a guide for performing a cultural assessment. When interviewing the patient, be flexible and ask only those questions that seem appropriate. Note that cultural assessment questions are broad and open ended; encourage the patient to express himself fully with descriptive responses.

Cultural affiliation
• I am interested in learning about your cultural heritage. Tell me about your cultural group. When did your ancestors come to North America and how many generations have lived here?

Health care beliefs and practices
• What does "care" mean to you? How do you and people in your community demonstrate care?
• What does "health" mean to you? What do you and others in your community do to stay healthy?
• Which types of food do you eat? Describe some of the customs surrounding meals in your culture.
• Describe your beliefs and practices regarding special life events such as birth and marriage.
• How are older people cared for in your culture?

Illness beliefs and customs
• Do people in your community uphold any religious or folk beliefs about treating illness? Do you agree with these beliefs? Does your culture have folk healers?
• Describe how illness is treated within your community. What are your own experiences in receiving treatment for illness?
• What are your experiences with health professionals? When do you consult with them?

Interpersonal relations
• Describe how people communicate with each other in your community. Consider such topics as the use of silence, proximity when talking, touching people, respect for people in authority, appropriate topics of conversation, and use of body and hands.
• Describe your family life.
• How do men and women interact with each other in your community? Does one sex dominate in social situations? How about at home?
• How do men and women meet in order to get married?
• What is your philosophy of raising children?

Performing a cultural assessment – *continued*

Spiritual practices
• Describe your religious beliefs and practices.
• Describe your feelings about life and death. What are your beliefs and practices related to the death of a loved one, and about souls, spirits, and the afterlife?
• What are the duties of men and women in your religion and place of worship?

World view and life-style
• What are the most important things in your life?
• Which languages are spoken in your home? Which languages do you understand and speak?
• What kinds of jobs do you and members of your family have? How do finances influence your way of life?
• What are your beliefs about the value of education? What kind of education have you received? What kind do you hope your children will receive?

inate his conversation. His language may seem so colloquial that it sounds like a foreign tongue. Here are some tips for working with a patient who speaks a different language or who possesses a different language skill level:
• Don't judge the patient's intellectual abilities or emotional status based on how he uses language.
• Don't assume that the patient is angry, aggressive, or hostile if he talks more loudly than is customary among North Americans of European descent.
• Use titles such as "Mr." or "Ms." unless you have established a first-name basis for the relationship.
• Don't attempt to imitate the patient's ethnic dialect; the patient may think you are mocking him or being condescending.
• Be attentive to the patient's nonverbal communication. Behavioral cues can help clarify confusing statements. Note the patient's appearance, how he moves, whether he maintains eye contact as well as his posture, facial expressions, gestures, and use of touch.
• Pay attention to the patient's communication preferences. For example, involve the patient's extended family in discussions or use oral rather than written teaching methods.
• Explain medical and nursing terms in simple, everyday words, and make sure that the patient understands your explanations.

• If you don't understand what the patient is saying, ask for clarification. Don't let excessive politeness or fear of embarrassment interfere with obtaining accurate assessment information.

Reviewing physiologic systems

Expect to review the patient's past and current physiologic status as part of the nursing health history. This will help you identify potential or undetected physiologic disorders. This review will include questions about the past and current function and maintenance of each body system. Try to avoid using complex technical language when asking questions. For most patients, you'll conduct the physiologic systems review in a head-to-toe sequence. (See *Assessing physiologic systems.*)

For a patient with a complex medical history, focus on the recent past. Ask, for example, "Have you had problems with your heart in the last year?" Review the patient's records, if available, to avoid duplicating information.

Performing the physiologic systems review for a patient with a complex medical history can be challenging. You may question which factors are significant or how the patient's signs and symptoms relate to the whole picture, and you may have difficulty keeping the patient focused on the system being assessed. Assessing each system just for the presence or absence of specific problems or symptoms is not adequate; you need to determine whether the problems affect the patient's ability to carry out activities of daily living. If so, you need to determine whether the patient can cope with the resulting complications.

When documenting the review of systems, note negative as well as positive findings. Don't be satisfied with vague answers, such as "a lot" or "a little." Try to obtain answers in sufficient detail.

Gathering data from secondary sources

Usually, information gathered directly from the patient — known as primary source data — is the most valuable because it reflects his situation most accurately. Additional data about a patient can be obtained from secondary sources, including family members, friends, and other members of the health care team. Written records — past clinical records, transfer summaries, and personal documents, such as a living will — also provide important information about the patient.

Secondary source information often provides an alternative to the viewpoints expressed by the patient. Sometimes, because

(Text continues on page 32.)

Assessing physiologic systems

When you assess a patient's physiologic status, be sure to ask appropriate questions about the function of each body system. Use the following phrases as guidelines for your questions.

General health status
- Unusual symptoms or problems
- Excessive fatigue
- Inability to tolerate exercise
- Number of colds or other minor illnesses per year
- Unexplained episodes of fever, weakness, or night sweats
- Impaired ability to carry out activities of daily living (ADL)

Skin, hair, and nails
- Known skin disease, such as psoriasis
- Itching
- Skin reaction to hot or cold weather
- Presence and location of scars, sores, or ulcers
- Presence and location of skin growths, such as warts, moles, tumors, or masses
- Color changes noted in any of the above lesions
- Changes in amount, texture, or character of hair
- Presence or development of baldness
- Hair care practices, including frequency of shampooing, perming, or hair coloring
- Changes in nail color or texture
- Excessive nail splitting, cracking, or breaking

Head and neck
- Lumps, bumps, or scars from old injuries
- Headaches (Perform a symptom analysis.)
- Recent head trauma, injury, or surgery
- Concussion or unconsciousness from head injury

- Dizzy spells or fainting
- Interference with normal range of motion
- Pain or stiffness (Perform a symptom analysis.)
- Swelling or masses
- Enlarged lymph nodes or glands

Nose and sinuses
- History of frequent nosebleeds
- History of allergies
- Postnasal drip
- Frequent sneezing
- Frequent nasal drainage (Note color, frequency, and amount.)
- Impaired ability to smell
- Pain over the sinuses
- History of nasal trauma or fracture
- Difficulty breathing through nostrils
- History of sinus infection and treatment received

Mouth and throat
- History of frequent sore throats — especially streptococcal (Perform a symptom analysis.)
- Current or past mouth lesions, such as abscesses, ulcers, or sores
- History of oral herpes infections
- Date and results of last dental examination
- Overall description of dental health
- Use of proper dental hygiene, including fluoride toothpaste (if applicable)
- Use of dentures or bridges
- Bleeding gums
- History of hoarseness
- Changes in voice quality
- Difficulty chewing or swallowing
- Changes in ability to taste

(continued)

Assessing physiologic systems – *continued*

Eyes
• Date and results of last vision examination
• Date and results of last check for glaucoma (for patients over age 50 or with a family history of glaucoma)
• History of eye infections or eye trauma
• Use of corrective lenses
• Itching, tearing, or discharge (Note color, amount, and time of occurrence as well as treatment received.)
• Eye pain
• Spots or floaters in visual field
• History of glaucoma or cataracts
• Blurred or double vision
• Unusual sensations, such as twitching
• Light sensitivity
• Swelling around eyes or eyelids
• Visual disturbances, such as rainbows around lights, blind spots, or flashing lights
• History of retinal detachment
• History of strabismus or amblyopia

Ears
• Date and results of last hearing evaluation
• Abnormal sensitivity to noise
• Ear pain
• Ringing or crackling in ears
• Recent changes in hearing ability
• Use of hearing aids
• History of ear infection
• History of vertigo
• Feeling of fullness in ear
• Ear care habits, including use of cotton-tipped applicators for ear wax removal
• Ear wax characteristics
• Number of ear infections per year (for pediatric patients)

Respiratory system
• History of asthma or other breathing problem (Perform a symptom analysis.)
• Chronic cough (Perform a symptom analysis.)
• History of coughing up blood
• Breathing problems after physical exertion
• Sputum production (Note color, odor, and amount.)
• Wheezing or noisy respirations
• History of pneumonia or bronchitis

Cardiovascular system
• History of chest pain
• History of palpitations
• History of heart murmur
• History of irregular pulse rates
• Hypertension
• Need to sit up to breathe, especially at night
• Coldness or numbness in extremities
• Color changes in fingers or toes
• Swelling or edema in extremities
• Leg pain when walking that's relieved by rest
• Hair loss on legs

Breasts
• Date and results of last breast examination (including mammography for women over age 40)
• Pattern of breast self-examination
• Breast pain, tenderness, or swelling (Perform a symptom analysis.)
• History of nipple changes or nipple discharge (Note color, odor, amount, and frequency.)
• History of breast-feeding

Gastrointestinal system
• Indigestion or pain associated with eating (Perform a symptom analysis.)
• History of ulcers
• History of vomiting blood
• Burning sensation in esophagus
• Frequent nausea and vomiting (Perform a symptom analysis.)
• History of liver disease

Assessing physiologic systems – *continued*

- History of jaundice
- History of gallbladder disease
- Abdominal swelling or ascites
- Changes in bowel elimination pattern
- Stool characteristics
- History of diarrhea or constipation
- History of hemorrhoids
- Use of digestive aids or laxatives
- Date and results of last fecal occult blood (Hemoccult) test (for patients over age 50)

Urinary system
- Painful urination
- Characteristics of urine
- Pattern of urination
- Hesitancy in starting urine stream
- Changes in urine stream
- History of kidney stones
- History of flank pain
- Blood in urine
- History of decreased or excessive urine output
- Dribbling, incontinence, or stress incontinence
- Frequent urination at night
- Difficulty with toilet training (for children)
- Bed-wetting (for children)
- History of bladder or kidney infections
- History of urinary tract infections

Female reproductive system
- Menstrual history, including age of onset, duration, and amount of flow
- Date of last menstrual period
- History of painful menstruation
- History of excessive menstrual bleeding
- History of missed periods
- History of bleeding between periods
- Date and results of last Pap test
- Obstetric history (for women of childbearing age), including number of

pregnancies, miscarriages, abortions, live births, and stillbirths
- Satisfaction with sexual relationships
- History of painful intercourse
- Contraceptive practices
- History of sexually transmitted disease
- Knowledge of how to prevent sexually transmitted diseases, including acquired immunodeficiency syndrome (AIDS)
- Problems with infertility

Male reproductive system
- Presence of penile lesions
- Presence of scrotal lesions
- Prostate problems
- Pattern of testicular self-examination
- Satisfaction with sexual relationships
- History of sexually transmitted disease
- Contraceptive practices
- Knowledge of how to prevent sexually transmitted diseases, including AIDS
- Concern about impotence
- Concern about sterility

Neurologic system
- History of fainting or loss of consciousness
- History of seizures or other nervous system problems; use of medication for seizure control
- History of cognitive disturbances, including recent or remote memory loss, hallucinations, disorientation, speech and language dysfunction, or inability to concentrate
- History of sensory disturbances, including tingling, numbness, or sensory loss
- History of motor problems, including problems with gait, balance, coordination, tremor, spasm, or paralysis
- Cognitive, sensory, or motor symptoms that interfere with ADL

(continued)

Assessing physiologic systems — *continued*

Musculoskeletal system
• History of fractures
• Muscle cramping, twitching, pain, or weakness (Perform a symptom analysis.)
• Limitations on walking, running, or participating in sports
• Joint swelling, redness, or pain
• Joint deformity
• Joint stiffness (Note time and duration.)
• Noise with joint movement
• Spinal deformity
• Chronic back pain (Perform a symptom analysis.)
• Musculoskeletal symptoms that interfere with ADL

Immune system and blood
• History of anemia
• History of bleeding tendencies
• History of easy bruising
• History of low platelet count
• History of becoming easily fatigued
• History of blood transfusion
• History of allergies, including eczema, hives, and itching

• Chronic clear nasal discharge
• Frequent sneezing
• Conjunctivitis
• Allergies that interfere with ADL
• Usual method of treating allergic symptoms
• History of frequent unexplained systemic infections
• Unexplained gland swelling

Endocrine system
• History of endocrine disease, such as thyroid problems, adrenal problems, or diabetes
• Unexplained changes in height or weight
• Increased thirst
• Increased urine output
• Increased food intake
• Heat or cold intolerance
• History of goiter
• Unexplained weakness
• Previous hormone therapy
• Changes in hair distribution
• Changes in skin pigmentation

of a patient's condition or age, secondary sources may be essential to establish a complete profile. For example, a young child or a patient who's profoundly confused may be unable to provide sufficient answers to your assessment questions.

Interviewing family members
Family members are often the most valuable source of secondary data. They may provide information about family dynamics, learning needs, and available support systems. You may also perform a family assessment to help ease family members' stress and help them cope with the patient's illness.

Consider asking the following questions as part of your family assessment:
• What is your relationship to the patient?

• What are the patient's major roles (such as breadwinner, homemaker, caregiver, and decision maker) within your family?

• Who will be assuming the patient's roles while he is hospitalized (spouse, parent, child, friend, neighbor)?

• Who assumes the role of head of your family?

• Who will act as family spokesperson? To whom shall I refer callers?

• Are any other factors (such as emotional, financial, child-rearing, other illness, or employment) putting stress on your family?

• Describe your family's decision-making patterns. Are major decisions made by spouses, parents, a family council, an extended family, or with outside resources (such as a minister)?

• Describe your family's support system (such as other relatives, neighbors, religious community, social groups, and friends).

• How would you say family members usually cope during a crisis? For example, do they become angry? Aggressive? Fearful? Sad? Withdrawn? Do they use regression or denial to cope?

• What kind of involvement does your family have with the community?

• What is the frequency and quality of communication among family members?

When interviewing family members, allow for open expression of feelings and avoid passing judgment. Maintain objectivity if family members appear to be in conflict. Keep in mind that family members may not always respond to the patient's needs as you would expect. (See *Assessing family relationships*, page 34.)

PERFORMING A PHYSICAL EXAMINATION
After the patient's health history, the next step in the assessment process is the physical examination. During the physical examination process, you collect objective data that may confirm or rule out suspicions raised during the health history. These findings will enable you to plan care and start teaching the patient about his condition. For example, an elevated blood pressure reading indicates that a patient may need a sodium-restricted diet and, possibly, instruction on controlling hypertension.

You need to be able to recognize deviations from the patient's normal physical and emotional characteristics. Explain to the

Assessing family relationships

Family members are best understood in the context of their relationships with each other. To cast light on how illness or injury has affected family relationships, consider asking questions that encourage family members to explore *differences* in their responses to the patient's illness. A sensitive assessment of family relationships can enable you to determine family needs more accurately.

Questions that foster insight

Carefully worded questions can provide the family with new information about itself. At best, new information and insight can help foster new ways of coping. The questions listed below are meant to provide examples of techniques for exploring family relationships. Of course, your questions must be tailored to the family's circumstances.

• Who in your family is handling the situation best?
• Who is most upset about your father's illness?
• What do you do when your mother shows she is upset?
• Who is more worried, your mother or your father?
• Who best understands the doctor's explanations of your father's illness?
• The last time your father was ill, who was most supportive?
• Who is closest to the patient?
• How is your family's response different now from the last time your father was in the intensive care unit?
• How did your brothers and sisters respond when first told about the illness?

   Throughout the assessment, show respect for family members' answers. Do not take sides; instead, focus on investigating and accepting the perception of each family member.

patient, clearly and concisely, what you are doing during the course of the examination.

   The scope of the physical examination depends on the patient's condition, the clinical setting, and the policies and procedures established by your health care facility. A routine neurologic examination on a medical-surgical unit, for example, may include assessing level of consciousness, orientation, muscle strength, and pupillary response. Abnormal findings would then lead you to perform a more in-depth assessment — an assessment that would be routine on a neurologic unit or critical care unit. (See *A quick review of the physical examination.*)

A quick review of the physical examination

The major components of the physical examination include the patient's height, weight, and vital signs as well as a review of the major body systems.

Respiratory system
Note the rate and rhythm of respirations, and auscultate the lung fields. Inspect the lips, mucous membranes, and nail beds. Also inspect any sputum, noting color, consistency, and other characteristics.

Cardiovascular system
Note the color and temperature of the extremities, and assess the peripheral pulses. Also check for edema and hair loss on the extremities. Inspect the neck veins and auscultate for heart sounds.

Neurologic system
Inspect the patient's head for evidence of trauma. Assess his level of consciousness, noting his orientation to person, place, and time and his ability to follow commands. Also assess pupillary reactions. Check extremities for movement and sensation.

Eyes, ears, nose, and throat
Assess the patient's ability to see objects (with or without corrective lenses). Also assess his ability to hear spoken words clearly. Inspect the eyes and ears for discharge; the nasal mucous membranes for dryness, irritation, and blood; and the teeth for cleanliness. Observe the condition of the oral mucous membranes, and palpate the lymph nodes in the neck.

GI system
Auscultate for bowel sounds in all quadrants. Note the presence of abdominal distention or ascites, and assess the condition of mucous membranes around the anus.

Musculoskeletal system
Assess the range of motion of major joints. Look for swelling at the joints and for contractures, muscle atrophy, or obvious deformity.

Genitourinary and reproductive systems
Note any bladder distention or incontinence. If indicated, inspect the genitalia for rashes, edema, or deformity. (Inspection of the genitalia may be waived at the patient's request or if no dysfunction was reported during the interview.) If indicated, inspect the genitalia for sexual maturity. Also examine the breasts, noting any abnormalities.

Integumentary system
Note any sores, lesions, scars, pressure ulcers, rashes, bruises, or petechiae. Also note the patient's skin turgor.

Choosing an examination method

The most commonly used methods for completing a total systematic physical assessment are head to toe and major body systems.

With the head-to-toe method, you systematically assess your patient — as the name suggests — beginning at the head and working toward the toes. Examine all parts of one body region before progressing to the next region to save time and energy for yourself and your patient. Proceed from left to right within each region so that you can make symmetrical comparisons. Don't examine the patient's left side from head to toe, then his right side.

The major-body-systems method involves systematically assessing your patient by examining each body system in priority order or in a predesignated sequence.

Both the head-to-toe and the major-body-systems methods are systematic and provide a logical, organized framework for collecting physical assessment data. They also provide the same information; therefore, neither is more correct than the other. So choose the method (or a variation of it) that works well for you and is appropriate for your patient population. Follow this routine whenever you assess a patient and try not to deviate from it.

When examining the patient, first determine whether his condition is life-threatening. Identifying the priority problems of a patient suffering from a life-threatening illness or injury — for example, severe trauma, heart attack, or GI hemorrhage — is essential to preserve his life and function and to prevent compounded damage.

Next, identify the patient population to which the patient belongs, and take the common characteristics of that population into account in choosing an examination method. For example, elderly or debilitated patients tire easily; for a patient in either category, you'd select a method that requires as few position changes as possible. Also, you'd probably defer parts of the examination to avoid tiring your patient.

View your patient as an integrated whole rather than as a collection of parts, regardless of the examination method you use. Remember, the integrity of a body region may reflect adequate functioning of many body systems, both inside and outside this particular region. For example, the integrity of the chest region may provide important clues about the functioning of the cardiovascular and respiratory systems. Similarly, the integrity of a body system may reflect adequate functioning of many body regions and of the various systems within these regions.

Chief complaint

You may want to plan your physical examination around your patient's chief complaint or concern. To do this, begin by examining the body system or region that corresponds to the chief complaint. This allows you to quickly identify priority problems and reassures your patient that you are paying attention to his primary reason for seeking health care.

Consider the following example. Your patient, Sarah Clemson, is a 65-year-old, active, well-nourished woman who appears younger than her chronological age. She complains of having difficulty breathing on exertion; she also has a dry, frequent, painful cough. Intermittent chills have persisted for 3 days. You'd record her vital signs as follows: temperature, 103° F (39.4° C); pulse rate, 106 beats/minute; respiratory rate, 29 to 30 breaths/minute; blood pressure, 128/82 mm Hg.

Because Mrs. Clemson's chief complaints are difficulty breathing, a cough, and chills, your physical examination would first focus on her respiratory system. You'd examine the patency of her airways, observe the color of her lips and extremities, and systematically palpate her lung fields for symmetry of expansion, crepitus, increased or decreased fremitus, and areas of tenderness. Then, after auscultating her lung fields for abnormal or adventitious sounds (such as crackles, rhonchi, or wheezing), you'd percuss her lung fields for increased or decreased resonance.

Next, you'd examine Mrs. Clemson's cardiovascular system, looking for further clues to the cause of her signs and symptoms. You'd inspect her neck veins for distention and her extremities for edema, venous engorgement, and pigmented areas. Then, you'd palpate her chest to see if you could feel the heart's apical impulse at the fifth intercostal space, in the midclavicular line. You'd also palpate for a precordial heave and for valvular thrills. After determining her apical pulse rate, you'd auscultate for any abnormal heart sounds.

At this point in the examination, you would probably be aware of Mrs. Clemson's level of consciousness, motor ability, and ability to use her muscles and joints. You probably wouldn't need to perform a more thorough musculoskeletal or neurologic examination. You would, however, proceed with an examination of her GI, genitourinary, and integumentary systems, modifying or shortening the examination sequences according to your findings and Mrs. Clemson's tolerance. If her signs and symptoms worsened during the examination, you'd interrupt the procedure to report her condition to her doctor. Then you'd plan to come back and finish the examination after her condition had stabilized.

Accurate and complete physical assessments depend on two interrelated elements. One is the use of sensory perception, by which you receive and perceive external stimuli. The other element is the conceptual process, by which you relate these stimuli to your knowledge base. By performing physical assessments systematically and efficiently instead of in a random or indiscriminate manner, you'll save time and identify priority problems quickly.

DOCUMENTING ASSESSMENT FINDINGS
All of the information you gather during assessment—initial general observations, the patient's history, and physical examination findings—must be recorded. Because assessment is a continuous process, you must also document your ongoing observations of the patient's condition for as long as he's under your care. The importance of this task cannot be overemphasized. Complete, accurate, and timely documentation of assessment data enables you and other health care providers to plan and coordinate quality patient care.

This section discusses tools and techniques for documenting the initial and ongoing assessments. It includes examples of formats that enable you to document assessment findings in a manner that accurately reflects the nursing process. You will also learn the advantages and disadvantages of different documentation styles.

Initial assessment
Depending on where you work, you may hear the initial assessment information referred to by any of several names, including the "nursing admission assessment" and the "nursing data base." Documentation styles and formats also vary, depending on the facility's policy and the patient population. You should be familiar with your facility's standards for documenting initial assessment findings appropriately.

Initial assessment findings are documented in one of three basic styles: narrative notes, standardized open-ended style, and standardized closed-ended style. Many assessment forms use a combination of all three styles.

Narrative notes
This documentation style consists of a handwritten account in paragraph form, summarizing information obtained by general observation, interview, and physical examination.

Although narrative notes allow you to list your findings in order of importance, they also pose problems. Frequently, the notes mimic the medical model by focusing on a review of body systems. They're also time-consuming—both to write and to read. Plus, narrative notes require you to remember and record all significant information in a detailed, logical sequence—often an unrealistic goal in today's hectic world of health care. Finally, difficulty in interpreting handwriting can easily lead to a misinterpretation of findings.

Standardized open-ended style
The typical "fill-in-the blanks" assessment form comes with preprinted headings and questions. This form saves you time in a couple of ways. Information is categorized under specific headings, so you can easily record and retrieve it. Also, the form can be completed using partial phrases and approved abbreviations. (See *Completing a standardized open-ended form*, page 40.)

Unfortunately, however, open-ended forms don't always provide the space or the instructions to encourage thorough descriptions. Thus, after the heading "type of dwelling," one nurse may write "apartment" whereas another may write "apartment with four-flight walk-up, without heat or hot water."

Nonspecific responses can, of course, lead to misinterpretation. For instance, a nurse may write that a patient performs a certain task "within normal limits." But unless normal limits have been defined, this notation is neither clear nor legally sound.

Standardized closed-ended style
This type of assessment form provides preprinted headings, checklists, and questions with specific responses. You simply check off the appropriate response. (See *Completing a standardized closed-ended form*, page 41.)

Besides saving time, the closed-ended form eliminates the problem of illegible handwriting and makes checking documented information easy. Plus, the form can be easily incorporated into most computerized systems. It also clearly establishes the type and amount of information required by
(Text continues on page 42.)

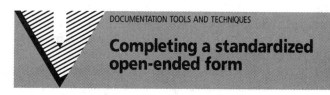

Completing a standardized open-ended form

At some health care facilities, you may use a standardized open-ended form to document initial assessment information. Here is a portion of such a form.

Reason for hospitalization _Attempted suicide_

Expected outcomes _Pt. won't harm self in hospital. Pt. recovers from suicidal episode. Pt. discusses feelings related to suicide attempt. Consultation with mental health professional arranged._

Last hospitalization
Date _5/25/93_ Reason _Severe depression_

Medical history _Physical health good._

Medications and allergies

Drug	Dosage	Time of last dose	Patient's statement of drug's purpose
imipramine	150mg. P.O.H.S	6/22/93 10 p.m.	"improve mood"

Allergy	Reaction
N/A	

DOCUMENTATION TOOLS AND TECHNIQUES

Completing a standardized closed-ended form

At some health care facilities, you may use a standardized closed-ended form to document initial assessment information. Here is a portion of such a form.

SELF-CARE ABILITY

Activity	1	2	3	4	5	6
Bathing			✓			
Cleaning			✓			
Climbing stairs			✓			
Cooking			✓			
Dressing and grooming			✓			
Eating and drinking	✓					
Moving in bed	✓					
Shopping			✓			
Toileting				✓		
Transferring			✓			
Walking			✓			
Other home functions			✓			

Key
1 Independent
2 Requires assistive device
3 Requires personal assistance
4 Requires personal assistance and assistive device
5 Dependent
6 Experienced change in last week

ASSISTIVE DEVICES
- ☑ Bedside commode
- ☐ Brace or splint
- ☐ Cane
- ☐ Crutches
- ☐ Feeding device
- ☐ Trapeze
- ☐ Walker
- ☐ Wheelchair
- ☐ Other
- ☐ None

ACTIVITY TOLERANCE
- ☐ Normal
- ☑ Weakness
- ☐ Dizziness
- ☐ Exertional dyspnea
- ☐ Dyspnea at rest
- ☐ Angina
- ☐ Pain at rest
- ☐ Oxygen needed
- ☐ Intermittent claudication
- ☐ Unsteady gait
- ☐ Other

REST PATTERN
Sleep habits
- ☑ Less than 8 hours
- ☐ 8 hours
- ☐ More than 8 hours
- ☐ Morning nap
- ☑ Afternoon nap

Sleep difficulties
- ☐ Insomnia
- ☑ Early awakening
- ☐ Unrefreshing sleep
- ☐ Nightmares
- ☐ None

the facility. And even though these forms commonly use non-specific terminology, such as "within normal limits" or "no alteration," guidelines clearly define these responses.

The closed-ended form also creates some problems. For instance, many of these forms provide no place to record relevant information that doesn't fit the preprinted choices. And the forms tend to be lengthy, especially when a hospital's policy calls for recording in-depth physical assessment data.

Alternative formats for documenting assessment

Historically, nursing assessment has followed a medical format, emphasizing the patient's initial symptoms and a comprehensive review of body systems. Although many health care facilities still use a medical format to organize their nursing assessment forms, some facilities have adopted formats that better reflect the nursing process.

Human response patterns

The North American Nursing Diagnosis Association (NANDA) has developed a classification system for nursing diagnoses based on human response patterns. Human response patterns are abstract categories — exchanging, communicating, relating, valuing, choosing, moving, perceiving, knowing, and feeling — used to classify each patient's actual or potential health problems. Although human response patterns were not originally intended to be used as an assessment framework, some documentation formats use them to organize assessment data. (For a more detailed explanation of NANDA's human response patterns, see Chapter 3, Nursing Diagnosis.)

When you use an assessment form organized by human response patterns, you can easily establish appropriate diagnoses while you record assessment data — especially if a listing of diagnoses is included with the form. The main drawback is that these forms tend to be lengthy. (See *Documenting human response patterns.)*

Functional health patterns

Some health care facilities organize their assessment data according to Gordon's functional health patterns. (See *Documenting functional health patterns,* page 44.) This system classifies nursing data according to the patient's ability to function independently.

Many nurses consider functional health patterns easier to understand and remember than human response patterns.

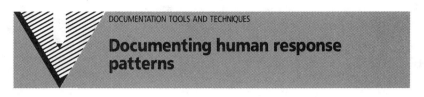

DOCUMENTATION TOOLS AND TECHNIQUES

Documenting human response patterns

Below you'll find one page of an assessment form that's organized by human response patterns. The sequence of response patterns varies among forms.

HEALTH HISTORY AND PHYSICAL EXAMINATION	
SUBJECTIVE DATA	**OBJECTIVE DATA**

SUBJECTIVE DATA

☑ Information from patient
☐ Information from significant other

OBJECTIVE DATA

MOVING

☐ Seizures
☑ Dizziness
☐ Paralysis
☐ Sleep difficulty
☐ Sleepwalking

Limits
☐ Walking
☐ Bathing
☐ Recreational
activities _____

Comments: *Pt suffered concussion 2 weeks ago. States dizziness started several days ago. Also reports fatigue.*

Joint mobility
☑ Moves all limbs
☐ Stiffness
☐ Equal grip
☐ Contractures
☐ Deformities
☐ Amputation

Gait
☐ Steady
☑ Unsteady
☐ Uses cane
☐ Uses walker
☐ Other: _____

Comments: *Pt describes feelings of "spinning around"*

RELATING AND CHOOSING

☑ Married   ☐ Widowed
☐ Separated   ☐ Single
☐ Divorced
Most supportive relatives or friends *wife*
☑ Alcohol use *social*
How much *12 oz. beer*
How often *about 2X/month*
☐ Substance abuse _____
Type _____
How much _____
How often _____

Observed behavior *anxious, moody*

Describe ability to comply with therapy (diet, medications, and so on) for chronic health problems (if applicable).

_____
N/A
_____

PERCEIVING AND COMMUNICATING

☐ Hearing impairment
☑ Visual impairment
Comments: *wears corrective lenses*

Describe pupils: *React to light*
☐ Blind _____
☐ Drainage from eyes _____
☐ Drainage from ears _____

Speech   ☐ Aphasic
☑ Normal   ☐ Slurred speech

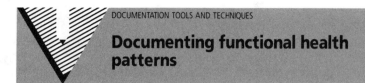

DOCUMENTATION TOOLS AND TECHNIQUES

Documenting functional health patterns

Below you'll see one page of an assessment form that's organized by functional health patterns. The sequence of health patterns varies among forms.

Date: *March 2, 1994*

COGNITION AND PERCEPTION

Mental status

☐ Alert and oriented   ☐ Unresponsive   ☐ Confused

☐ Lethargic   ☐ Aphasic   ☐ Periodically

☑ Depressed   ☐ Combative   ☐ At night

     ☐ At all times

Vision

☐ Normal   ☐ Eyeglasses   ☐ Left cataract   ☐ Left blind

☐ Left impaired   ☑ Contacts   ☐ Right cataract   ☐ Right blind

☐ Right impaired   ☐ Prosthesis   ☐ Glaucoma

Hearing

☑ Normal   ☐ Left impaired   ☐ Left deaf   ☐ Tinnitus

☐ Hearing aid   ☐ Right impaired   ☐ Right deaf

Speech

☐ Normal   ☐ Garbled   ☐ Language barrier

☐ Slurred   ☐ Expressive aphasia   Language spoken *English*

Pain

☐ None   ☐ Acute   ☑ Chronic

Describe pain and its management: *Pt. describes "dull headache"; takes Tylenol*

COPING AND STRESS TOLERANCE

Describe patient's concerns about hospitalization.

Anxious about possible diagnosis.

Identify coping methods used previously.

Relied on husband and neighbors

Describe any major loss or change in the last year.

Recently divorced; just reentered job market

VALUES AND BELIEFS

☐ Cultural practices _____

Religion

☐ Catholic   ☐ Jewish   ☐ Other _____

☑ Protestant   ☐ None

Generally, assessment forms based on functional health patterns are easier and less time-consuming to complete.

Ongoing assessment

Your assessment of a patient is a continuous process; it begins when you first encounter the patient and continues throughout his hospitalization. Reassessment lets you evaluate the effectiveness of your nursing interventions and determine your patient's progress toward the expected outcomes. It helps you determine if you need to revise, extend, or discontinue nursing interventions. You may also identify other health problems that develop as a result of illness, hospitalization, or treatment.

Flow sheets

You'll usually document ongoing assessment data on flow sheets or in narrative notes on the patient's progress report. Ideally, you should use flow sheets to document all routine assessment data and nursing interventions. That way, you can shorten the narrative notes to include only information regarding the patient's progress toward achieving expected outcomes and any unplanned assessments. (See *Completing an assessment flow sheet,* page 46.)

Flow sheets come in many varieties, including temperature graphs and intake and output forms. When used to record routine assessment data, flow sheets can be a quick and consistent way to highlight trends in the patient's condition. A flow sheet for documenting information about a patient's skin integrity, for instance, will clearly show the progression of any pressure ulcers or reddened areas.

Because flow sheets are legally accepted components of the patient's clinical record, they must be documented correctly. Give yourself enough time to evaluate each piece of information on the flow sheet. Keep in mind that it must accurately reflect the patient's current status.

In some cases, you'll find that recording only the information requested on a flow sheet won't be sufficient to give a complete picture of the patient's status. When this occurs, record additional information in the space provided on the flow sheet.

If additional information isn't necessary, draw a line through the space. Doing so indicates that, in your judgment, further information isn't required. If your flow sheet doesn't have additional space and you need to record more information, use the nurses' progress notes.

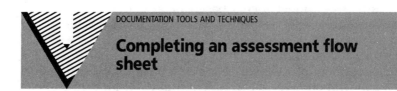

Completing an assessment flow sheet

The sample below shows a portion of an assessment flow sheet.

ASSESSMENT FLOW SHEET

Date _____ 7/10/93 _____

DIET	
Meal	**Amount eaten**
Breakfast	100 %
Lunch	90 %
Dinner	90 %

☑ By himself
☐ With help
☐ With NG tube

HYGIENE	7-3	3-11	11-7
By himself	SK	JM	
With some help			
With complete help			
Shower			
Oral care	SK	JM	
P.M. care		JM	
Catheter care			

ACTIVITY & REST			
On complete bed rest			
Turn q 2 hr			
OOB (chair)			
BRP	SK	JM	BB
Walking	SK	JM	BB

ELIMINATION			
Normal voiding	SK	JM	BB
Has catheter			
Incontinent			
Bowel movement			

PULSE	7-3	3-11	11-7
Regular	SK	JM	BB
Irregular			
Strong	SK	JM	BB
Weak			

MUSCULOSKELETAL			
Moves all limbs	SK	JM	BB
Weak			
Paralyzed			
Paresthetic			

RESPIRATORY			
Respirations			
Within normal limits	SK	JM	BB
Shallow			
Deep			
Labored			
Respiratory rate			
Within normal limits	SK	JM	BB
Slow			
Rapid			
Breath sounds			
Clear	SK	JM	BB
Moist			
Wheezing			
Coughing			

SKIN			
Temperature			
Cool			
Warm	SK	JM	BB
Hot			

A final caution: Avoid judgments and conclusions

The importance of avoiding judgments and conclusions in your assessment and documentation can best be illustrated by example. Consider this story from a registered nurse at a large city hospital:

When the ambulance crew brought Brandon Morrison, age 19, into the emergency department, they could barely control him. He was struggling and shouting that spiders were crawling on his body.

Brandon was a known I.V. drug user, and our staff had just treated him a month earlier for an overdose. Assuming he'd overdosed again, we restrained him, took his vital signs, and then drew blood for a toxicology study.

When the test results came back an hour later, I was astonished. Brandon's serum glucose level was only 26 mg/dl. After more extensive testing, we realized that besides having a drug problem, he also had diabetes.

We quickly started an I.V. line with dextrose 50%, and within minutes, Brandon was awake, oriented, and cooperative. But if we'd delayed treatment any longer, he might have suffered permanent brain damage.

During the assessment, keep your observations objective and don't draw conclusions. Initial conclusions are frequently wrong because they're based on too little evidence. To document properly, you should record just the facts.

KEY POINTS

• Assessment is the first and most critical step in the nursing process; it yields all the data you need to carry out the nursing process and deliver the best possible patient care.
• The nursing health history is distinguished by its holistic focus on the human response to illness, whereas the medical history is designed to guide diagnosis and treatment of illness.
• An assessment requires consideration of subjective and objective information. Subjective information represents the patient's perception of a problem. Objective information is data you can observe or measure and can verify.
• Assessment is an ongoing process; it begins when you first encounter the patient and continues throughout his hospitalization. All information gathered during assessment—initial observations, patient history, physical examination findings,

and ongoing observations — must be documented thoroughly and accurately.

• When eliciting subjective information during the patient interview, ask questions that encourage that patient to describe the nature of his complaint in detail.

• When recording objective data, write down facts, using measurements when possible. Avoid vague terms such as "large" or "small." Avoid documenting judgments and conclusions.

• Primary source data — information obtained from the patient — usually is the most important because it most accurately reflects the patient's situation. Secondary sources, such as family members and past clinical records, supplement primary data. These sources can be essential when a patient's condition makes it difficult to gather adequate primary data.

• Learning to use effective communication techniques can help to ensure a successful patient interview. Such techniques include offering general leads, rephrasing the essence of the patient's comments, focusing the discussion, encouraging the patient to express himself, clarifying vague or confusing remarks, stating observations about the patient's behavior, and summarizing each health history component.

• Two methods of performing the physical examination are the head-to-toe method and the major-body-systems method. Regardless of which method you use, you should view the patient as an integrated whole rather than a collection of parts.

• The patient's chief complaint often provides a focal point around which to plan the physical examination. Begin by examining the body system or region that corresponds to the chief complaint.

• Initial assessment findings are documented in one of three basic styles: narrative notes (handwritten account), standardized open-ended style (fill-in-the-blanks), and standardized closed-ended style (checklist).

• Historically, nursing assessments have followed a medical format. Today, many health care facilities are adopting formats that more accurately reflect the nursing process, such as NANDA's human response patterns or Gordon's functional health patterns.

• Ongoing assessment enables you to evaluate the effectiveness of your nursing interventions and determine your patient's progress toward expected outcomes. Usually, you'll document ongoing assessment data on flow sheets or in narrative notes on the patient's progress report.

SELF-TEST

1. Which statement describes the nursing health history most accurately?

   a. The nursing history is designed to guide diagnosis and treatment of the illness.
   b. The nursing history is a follow-up to the medical history.
   c. The nursing history is taken after you perform your physical examination of the patient.
   d. The nursing history is distinguished by its holistic focus on the human response to illness.

2. The three phases of the nursing health history interview include:

   a. introduction, body, and closure.
   b. physical examination, data analysis, and expected outcomes.
   c. data gathering, introduction, and closure.
   d. physical examination, interview, and planning care.

3. Which statement most accurately describes the difference between subjective and objective data?

   a. Subjective data are used when formulating nursing diagnoses; objective data are used by doctors when formulating medical diagnoses.
   b. Subjective information represents the patient's perceptions; objective information can be observed or measured and can be verified.
   c. Obtaining accurate objective data is the most important part of the nursing health history. If you collect detailed and complete objective data, you won't need subjective information.
   d. Objective and subjective data are essentially the same.

4. Which of the following interview techniques is appropriate?

   a. sharing experiences with the patient and giving advice
   b. avoiding general questions because responses to them are not specific enough to be of value
   c. allowing the patient to digress to promote uninhibited expression of thoughts and feelings

d. remaining silent for short periods to reduce anxiety and give the patient a chance to organize his thoughts

5. Which of the following actions is *incorrect* when trying to communicate with a hearing-impaired or elderly patient?

a. touching the patient gently on the arm to let him know you're in the room

b. making sure he has his eyeglasses on when speaking to him

c. beginning your talk with the patient by stating the subject of the conversation

d. not rushing the patient when he is trying to express himself

6. Which of the following actions is *incorrect* when assessing a patient who speaks in an unfamiliar language or dialect?

a. not assuming the patient is angry if he talks more loudly than is usual among Americans

b. using the title "Mr." or "Ms." unless you've established a first-name basis for the relationship

c. speaking in the patient's ethnic dialect to put him at ease

d. asking a friend or family member to serve as a translator

7. The difference between an open-ended and a closed-ended assessment form is:

a. an open-ended form is designed for documenting the nursing health history; a closed-ended form is designed for use in medical assessments.

b. an open-ended form is a "fill-in-the-blanks" form; a closed-ended form has checklists.

c. an open-ended form is used in the initial assessment; a closed-ended form is used in ongoing assessment.

d. a closed-ended form is used in the initial assessment; an open-ended form is used in reassessments.

8. You obtain subjective information by:

a. observing your patient.

b. performing a physical examination.

c. listening to your patient's descriptions of his symptoms.

d. all of the above.

9. The primary source of assessment information is:

a. the patient's family.
b. the patient.
c. the patient's previous clinical records.
d. all of the above.

10. The North American Nursing Diagnosis Association bases its classification system for nursing diagnoses on:

a. the medical model.
b. human response patterns.
c. functional health patterns.
d. the patient's ability to function independently.

11. When deciding on a method of physical examination, you should:

a. consider whether the patient's condition is life-threatening.
b. consider the characteristics of your patient population.
c. try to use the same examination routine all the time.
d. all of the above.

(For answers with rationales, turn to page 260.)

FURTHER READINGS

Alfaro, R. *Applying Nursing Diagnosis and Nursing Process: A Step-by-Step Guide*, 2nd ed. Philadelphia: J.B. Lippincott Co., 1989.

Better Documentation. Clinical Skillbuilders Series. Springhouse, Pa.: Springhouse Corp., 1992.

Brown, M. "How Do You Spell Assessment?" *American Journal of Nursing* 91(9):55-56, September 1991.

Doenges, M.E., and Moorhouse, M.F. *Application of Nursing Process and Nursing Diagnosis: An Interaction Text*. Philadelphia: F.A. Davis Co., 1992.

Hartman, D., and Knudson, J. "Documentation: A Nursing Data Base for Initial Patient Assessment," *Oncology Nursing Forum* 18(1):125-30, January-February 1991.

Haselfeld, D. "Patient Assessment: Conducting an Effective Interview," *AORN Journal* 52(3):551-57, September 1990.

Iyer, P.W., et al. *Nursing Process and Nursing Diagnosis,* 2nd ed. Philadelphia: W.B. Saunders Co., 1991.

Jablonski, R.A.S. "Remember the Person Attached to the Ventilator," *Nursing92* 22(4):67-70, April 1992.

Loos, F., and Bell, J.M. "Circular Questions: A Family Interviewing Strategy," *Dimensions in Critical Care Nursing* 9(1):46-53, January-February 1990.

McConnell, E.A. "Do You Really Know What's Troubling Your Patient?" *Nursing90* 20(2):43, February 1990.

Mikhail, J.N. "Developing a Family Assessment and Intervention Protocol," *Critical Care Nurse* 8(3):114-18, May 1988.

Morton, P.G. *Health Assessment in Nursing,* 2nd ed. Springhouse, Pa.: Springhouse Corp., 1993.

Rosenbaum, J.N. "A Cultural Assessment Guide: Learning Cultural Sensitivity," *Canadian Nurse* 87(4):32-33, April 1991.

Sparks, S.M., and Taylor, C.M. *Nursing Diagnosis Reference Manual,* 2nd ed. Springhouse, Pa.: Springhouse Corp., 1993.

NURSING DIAGNOSIS

Of all the nursing process steps, nursing diagnosis remains the most controversial. Although the concept of nursing diagnosis has gained acceptance in nursing schools and textbooks, it has been less readily accepted in clinical practice. That's because many nurses and other health care professionals have trouble understanding the purpose of nursing diagnoses and separating nursing diagnoses from medical diagnoses. What's more, some nurses are reluctant to take the time to develop nursing diagnoses for each patient, and others complain that nursing diagnosis terminology is confusing.

However, understanding nursing diagnoses and learning how to apply them in clinical practice is important. After all, nursing diagnosis defines the practice of nursing: It spells out what nurses do and makes clear how nursing practice is distinct from the work of doctors and other health professionals.

Nursing diagnoses are likely to become increasingly important in clinical practice, especially as more health care facilities adopt computerized information systems. After all, nursing diagnoses are standardized labels that allow accurate recording of nursing activities in a computer data base. Companies that design and sell hospital information systems almost always incorporate nursing diagnoses into their software packages.

Careful identification and accurate documentation of nursing diagnoses can significantly improve continuity of care. In effect, each nurse who cares for the patient can know exactly what his problems are and can better prepare to meet his nursing needs.

Reading this chapter will enable you to see through the confusion surrounding nursing diagnoses. You may find that developing a nursing diagnosis does take some practice but that it's not difficult. The chapter begins with a definition of nursing diagnosis, goes on to distinguish the concept from medical diagnosis, and provides guidelines for using nursing diagnoses in clinical practice. You'll also find a short history of the nursing diagnosis movement, including an introduction to the North American Nursing Diagnosis Association (NANDA). At the end of the chapter, a series of case studies illustrates how to use nursing diagnoses in various clinical settings.

WHAT IS A NURSING DIAGNOSIS?

In 1990, NANDA adopted the following definition of a nursing diagnosis:

A nursing diagnosis is a clinical judgment about individual, family, or community responses to actual or potential health problems or life processes. Nursing diagnoses provide the basis for the selection of nursing interventions to achieve outcomes for which the nurse is accountable.

This definition includes three key points:

• When you formulate a nursing diagnosis, you are making a judgment about the patient's response to health problems or life processes.

• When planning care, you select nursing interventions to address the human responses described in the nursing diagnosis.

• You are accountable for achieving patient outcomes that are derived from the nursing diagnosis.

Fostering a holistic approach to care

Before the development of nursing diagnoses, nurses used experience and intuition along with knowledge of medical diagnoses to plan patient care. As a profession, nursing became distinguished for its focus on caring for the whole patient—instead of just reacting to a disorder. Nursing diagnoses help reinforce the nursing outlook on patient care.

Becoming adept at using nursing diagnoses will help you to shift your focus from treating signs and symptoms of medical disorders to caring for the whole patient. Nursing diagnoses encourage you to help the patient cope with his current state of health rather than focus entirely on curing disease. This approach to care maximizes the chances of a positive outcome regardless of the course of the patient's illness.

Nursing diagnoses do not catalog every nursing task. Rather, they describe the range of patient problems and needs amenable to nursing intervention. The emphasis on patient responses to health problems and life processes has helped to define the area of health care specific to nursing. (See *Not a nursing diagnosis*.)

Not a nursing diagnosis

Keep in mind that a nursing diagnosis is a statement of a health problem that a nurse is licensed to treat—a problem for which you'll assume responsibility for therapeutic decisions and accountability for the outcomes. A nursing diagnosis is *not:*
• a diagnostic test ("schedule for cardiac angiography")
• a piece of equipment ("set up intermittent suction apparatus")
• a problem with equipment ("the patient has trouble using a commode")
• a nurse's problem with a patient ("Mr. Jones is a difficult patient; he's rude and won't take his medication")
• a nursing goal ("encourage fluids up to 2,000 ml per day")
• a nursing need ("I have to get through to the family that they must accept their father's dying")
• a medical diagnosis ("cervical cancer") or treatment ("catheterize after each voiding for residual urine").

Medical vs. nursing diagnoses

To better understand nursing diagnoses, consider how nursing diagnoses are distinct from medical diagnoses:
• Medical diagnoses are labels for diseases or organ dysfunctions. In contrast, nursing diagnoses are labels for human responses to actual or potential health problems or life processes.
• Medical diagnoses usually describe the patient's illness without considering his relationship to family or community. In contrast, nursing diagnoses may be used to describe the patient's relationship with family and community. Specific nursing diagnoses, such as *altered family processes,* describe the family as a functioning unit.
• Medical diagnoses remain the same until the disease or dysfunction is cured. Nursing diagnoses may change hourly, daily, monthly—whenever the patient's response pattern changes.
• Medical diagnoses address pathophysiologic changes in the body. Nursing diagnoses address the patient's behavioral and physiologic responses to health problems or life processes.

You can use nursing diagnoses to describe physiologic disturbances. Various nursing diagnoses (for example, *decreased cardiac output, altered tissue perfusion, fluid volume deficit,* and *dysfunctional ventilatory weaning response*) describe physiologic problems that nurses treat independently or in collaboration with the medical staff.

Distinguishing between medical and nursing diagnoses

In the chart below, each synopsis describes related assessment findings for a patient. Reviewing the corresponding medical and nursing diagnoses points out the distinction in how each discipline interprets this information.

SYNOPSIS	MEDICAL DIAGNOSIS	NURSING DIAGNOSES
For 5 consecutive days, Mary Wilson, age 26, has experienced sporadic abdominal cramps of increasing intensity. Most recently, the pain has been accompanied by vomiting and a slight fever. When you examine Mary, you find rebound tenderness and muscle guarding.	Appendicitis	• Pain related to unknown etiology • Fluid volume deficit related to vomiting • Anxiety related to unknown abdominal condition
Frank Smith, age 67, complains of "stubborn, old muscles." He has difficulty walking, as you can see by his shuffling gait. During the interview, Mr. Smith speaks in a monotone and seems very depressed. Physical examination shows a pill-rolling hand tremor. Laboratory tests reveal a decrease in dopamine level.	Parkinson's disease	• Impaired physical mobility related to decreased muscle control • Body image disturbance related to physical alterations • Knowledge deficit related to lack of information about progressive nature of illness
During an extensive bout with respiratory tract infections, Tom Bradley, age 7, complains of throbbing ear pain. Tom's mother notes his hearing difficulty and his fear that he won't get better. On inspection, his tympanic membrane appears red and bulging.	Acute suppurative otitis media	• Pain related to lack of knowledge of pain management techniques • Fear related to lack of understanding of disease process • High risk for sensory or perceptual alteration (auditory)

• Finally, formulating a medical diagnosis is within the legally permissible scope of medical practice; formulating a nursing diagnosis is within the legally permissible scope of nursing practice. (See *Distinguishing between medical and nursing diagnoses*.)

UNDERSTANDING N.A.N.D.A. TAXONOMY

In an effort to make nursing diagnoses consistent, several organizations have developed standardized lists, which are used by a growing number of health care facilities. NANDA's list is the most widely accepted. (See *History of nursing diagnosis*, pages 58 and 59.)

Originally, NANDA listed nursing diagnoses alphabetically. In an effort to make the list easier to use, a committee of nurse theorists devised a classification system—the NANDA taxonomy—that categorizes nursing diagnoses according to the following human response patterns: exchanging, communicating, relating, valuing, choosing, moving, perceiving, knowing, and feeling. (See *Understanding human response patterns*, pages 60 and 61.)

Human response patterns do not form a framework for patient assessment or a specific nursing theory. They're simply a way to organize nursing diagnoses.

In the NANDA taxonomy, each nursing diagnosis is listed under the most appropriate heading and assigned a classification number. The numbers have no inherent order; they're assigned individually as diagnoses are approved. The number of digits assigned is related to the level of abstraction of the nursing diagnosis (more specific diagnoses are assigned longer numbers). The numbers are intended to facilitate computerization of the taxonomy. (See *NANDA's Taxonomy I Revised*, pages 62 and 63.)

A UNIVERSAL STANDARD?

NANDA members have translated the NANDA taxonomy into a version compatible with the format of the *International Classification of Diseases (ICD)*, published by the World Health Organization (WHO). *ICD* codes are used worldwide to compile statistics on the use of health care resources and to report information on morbidity and mortality rates. In the United States, doctors use *ICD* codes to obtain payment from third-party payers, such as insurance companies and the federal government. (See *NANDA taxonomy: The ICD translation*, pages 64 and 65.)

NANDA and the American Nurses' Association have submitted the *ICD* version of the taxonomy to WHO and to the publishers of the American version of the *ICD*, commonly known as *ICD-CM*. A decision about whether to include nursing diagnoses in the *ICD-CM* is expected in 1993 or 1994.

Formal classification of nursing diagnoses within the *ICD* framework could have a dramatic effect on nursing practice. It could lead to the development of an international nursing

(Text continues on page 66.)

History of nursing diagnosis

Originally, the nursing process consisted of only four distinct phases: assessment (which included diagnosis), planning, implementation, and evaluation. However, within the past two decades, diagnosis has become a distinct part of the process. Several events encouraged this important development.

The birth of NANDA
In the early 1970s, nurses Kristine M. Gebbie and Mary Ann Lavin participated in a project that involved computerizing nursing care information. They were asked to organize this information so that it could be retrieved easily from a computer data base and to code data so that nursing care could be distinguished from that provided by other health care personnel.

While working on this project, Gebbie and Lavin realized that resources for validating and quantifying nursing care were highly inadequate. This experience led them to organize the first National Conference Group for the Classification of Nursing Diagnoses in 1973. Participants in this group worked on identifying, developing, and classifying nursing diagnoses at a series of national conferences. At the fifth conference in 1982, the group adopted its official name—the North American Nursing Diagnosis Association (NANDA). Since then, NANDA has held biennial conferences; its most recent conference took place in San Diego in April 1992.

Today, members of NANDA collaborate with the American Nurses' Association (ANA) and other nursing specialty organizations to test and refine approved diagnoses and to identify, develop, test, and classify new diagnoses. They also are standardizing the entire classification system to make it compatible with computerized health care data bases.

Highlights
The following are highlights from the history of nursing diagnosis.

YEAR	EVENT
1950	R. Louise McManus first describes diagnosis as a function of nursing in the publication *Assumptions of the Functions of Nursing*.
1955	Lydia Hall first describes the nursing process in the article "Quality of Nursing Care: An Address to the New Jersey League for Nursing" in *Public Health News*.
1960	Faye G. Abdellah becomes the first person to classify nursing problems in the publication *Patient Centered Approach to Nursing*.
1967	Helen Yura and Mary Walsh publish the first book on the nursing process, *The Nursing Process: Assessing, Planning, Implementing, Evaluating*. Note that this book uses a four-step approach.

History of nursing diagnosis – *continued*

YEAR	EVENT
1973	The ANA publishes *Standards of Nursing Practice;* standard II specifically recognizes nursing diagnosis as a distinct phase of nursing.
	First conference on the classification of nursing diagnoses.
1975	Mary Mundinger and Grace Jauron become the first to separate nursing diagnosis from the assessment step of the nursing process to create a five-step approach. They publish their work in the article "Developing a Nursing Diagnosis" in *Nursing Outlook.*
	Second conference on the classification of nursing diagnoses.
1978	Third conference on the classification of nursing diagnoses; nurse theorists begin developing a framework for classifying nursing diagnoses.
1980	Fourth conference on the classification of nursing diagnoses.
	The ANA publishes *Nursing: A Social Policy Statement,* which defines nursing as the diagnosis and treatment of human responses to health problems.
1982	Fifth conference on the classification of nursing diagnoses; nurse theorists submit proposed taxonomic structure; NANDA is officially organized.
1983	Judith J. Warren demonstrates the use of nursing diagnosis in establishing accountability measures in nursing in the article "Accountability and Nursing Diagnosis" in the *Journal of Nursing Administration.*
1984	Sixth NANDA conference.
1986	Seventh NANDA conference. NANDA endorses *Taxonomy I* for development and testing.
1987	First international nursing diagnosis conference in Calgary, Canada.
	The ANA endorses NANDA as the organization responsible for classifying nursing diagnoses.
1988	Eighth NANDA conference.
1990	Ninth NANDA conference. NANDA publishes *Taxonomy I Revised.*
1991	The Joint Commission on Accreditation of Healthcare Organizations (JCAHO) incorporates the concept of nursing diagnosis into its revised standards for nursing care; JCAHO standards require that each patient's care be based on nursing diagnoses (or patient problems) identified by a registered nurse.
	The ANA publishes its revised *Standards of Clinical Nursing Practice,* which continues to recognize nursing diagnosis as a separate step in the nursing process.
1992	Tenth NANDA Conference.

Understanding human response patterns

NANDA uses nine human response patterns as a framework for organizing nursing diagnoses. Each time a new nursing diagnosis is added to the NANDA taxonomy, it is placed within the most appropriate pattern. Placement of diagnoses is based on the correlation between the definition of the diagnosis and the definition of the response pattern.

PATTERN AND DEFINITION	DIAGNOSES INCLUDED IN PATTERN
Exchanging • Giving, relinquishing, or losing something while receiving something in return • Substituting one element for another • The reciprocal act of giving and receiving	Altered nutrition; high risk for altered nutrition; high risk for infection; high risk for altered body temperature; hypothermia; hyperthermia; ineffective thermoregulation; dysreflexia; constipation; perceived constipation; colonic constipation; diarrhea; incontinence (bowel, stress, reflex, urge, functional, total); altered urinary elimination; urinary retention; altered tissue perfusion; fluid volume excess; fluid volume deficit; high risk for fluid volume deficit; decreased cardiac output; impaired gas exchange; ineffective airway clearance; ineffective breathing pattern; inability to sustain spontaneous ventilation; dysfunctional ventilatory weaning response; high risk for injury; high risk for suffocation; high risk for poisoning; high risk for trauma; high risk for aspiration; high risk for disuse syndrome; altered protection; impaired tissue integrity; altered oral mucous membrane; impaired skin integrity; high risk for impaired skin integrity
Communicating • Conversing • Transmitting thoughts, feelings, or information verbally or nonverbally	Impaired verbal communication
Relating • Establishing a link with a person, place, or thing • Establishing bonds • Connecting or associating with others	Impaired social interaction; social isolation; altered role performance; altered parenting; high risk for altered parenting; sexual dysfunction; altered family processes; caregiver role strain; high risk for caregiver role strain; parental role conflict; altered sexuality patterns
Valuing • Being concerned about, caring • Noting the worth of something • Forming a favorable opinion of a person or thing	Spiritual distress (distress of the human spirit)

Understanding human response patterns — *continued*

PATTERN AND DEFINITION	DIAGNOSES INCLUDED IN PATTERN
Choosing • Selecting between alternatives • Selecting or exercising preference in regard to a matter in which one is a free agent • Determining in favor of a course • Deciding in accordance with inclinations	Ineffective individual coping; impaired adjustment; defensive coping; ineffective denial; ineffective family coping (disabling, compromised); family coping: potential for growth; ineffective management of therapeutic regimen (individual); noncompliance; decisional conflict; health-seeking behaviors
Moving • Changing the place or position of a body or any part of the body • Placing or keeping something in motion • Provoking an excretion or discharge • Taking action • Experiencing the urge to do something	Impaired physical mobility; high risk for peripheral neurovascular dysfunction; activity intolerance; fatigue; high risk for activity intolerance; sleep pattern disturbance; diversional activity deficit; impaired home maintenance management; altered health maintenance; feeding self-care deficit; impaired swallowing; ineffective breast-feeding; interrupted breast-feeding; effective breast-feeding; ineffective infant feeding pattern; bathing or hygiene self-care deficit; dressing or grooming self-care deficit; toileting self-care deficit; altered growth and development; relocation stress syndrome
Perceiving • Becoming aware through the senses • Apprehending what is not open or present to observation • Absorbing fully and adequately	Body image disturbance; self-esteem disturbance; chronic low self-esteem; situational low self-esteem; personal identity disturbance; sensory or perceptual alterations; unilateral neglect; hopelessness; powerlessness
Knowing • Recognizing or acknowledging a thing or a person • Becoming familiar with facts by experience or through information or report • Becoming cognizant of something through observation or inquiry or through receiving information • Developing understanding	Knowledge deficit; altered thought processes
Feeling • Experiencing a sensation, apprehension, or sense • Being consciously or emotionally affected by a fact, event, or state	Pain; chronic pain; dysfunctional grieving; anticipatory grieving; high risk for violence; high risk for self-mutilation; posttrauma response; rape-trauma syndrome (compound reaction, silent reaction); anxiety; fear

NANDA's *Taxonomy I Revised*

NANDA's *Taxonomy I Revised*, organized around nine human response patterns, is the currently accepted classification system for nursing diagnoses. The complete taxonomic structure is listed below.

Pattern 1
Exchanging: A human response pattern involving mutual giving and receiving

1.1.2.1	Altered nutrition: More than body requirements
1.1.2.2	Altered nutrition: Less than body requirements
1.1.2.3	Altered nutrition: High risk for more than body requirements
1.2.1.1	High risk for infection
1.2.2.1	High risk for altered body temperature
1.2.2.2	Hypothermia
1.2.2.3	Hyperthermia
1.2.2.4	Ineffective thermoregulation
1.2.3.1	Dysreflexia
1.3.1.1	Constipation
1.3.1.1.1	Perceived constipation
1.3.1.1.2	Colonic constipation
1.3.1.2	Diarrhea
1.3.1.3	Bowel incontinence
1.3.2	Altered urinary elimination
1.3.2.1.1	Stress incontinence
1.3.2.1.2	Reflex incontinence
1.3.2.1.3	Urge incontinence
1.3.2.1.4	Functional incontinence
1.3.2.1.5	Total incontinence
1.3.2.2	Urinary retention
1.4.1.1	Altered (specify type) tissue perfusion (renal, cerebral, cardiopulmonary, gastrointestinal, peripheral)
1.4.1.2.1	Fluid volume excess
1.4.1.2.2.1	Fluid volume deficit
1.4.1.2.2.2	High risk for fluid volume deficit
1.4.2.1	Decreased cardiac output
1.5.1.1	Impaired gas exchange
1.5.1.2	Ineffective airway clearance
1.5.1.3	Ineffective breathing pattern
1.5.1.3.1	Inability to sustain spontaneous ventilation

1.5.1.3.2	Dysfunctional ventilatory weaning response
1.6.1	High risk for injury
1.6.1.1	High risk for suffocation
1.6.1.2	High risk for poisoning
1.6.1.3	High risk for trauma
1.6.1.4	High risk for aspiration
1.6.1.5	High risk for disuse syndrome
1.6.2	Altered protection
1.6.2.1	Impaired tissue integrity
1.6.2.1.1	Altered oral mucous membrane
1.6.2.1.2.1	Impaired skin integrity
1.6.2.1.2.2	High risk for impaired skin integrity

Pattern 2
Communicating: A human response pattern involving sending messages

2.1.1.1	Impaired verbal communication

Pattern 3
Relating: A human response pattern involving establishing bonds

3.1.1	Impaired social interaction
3.1.2	Social isolation
3.2.1	Altered role performance
3.2.1.1.1	Altered parenting
3.2.1.1.2	High risk for altered parenting
3.2.1.2.1	Sexual dysfunction
3.2.2	Altered family processes
3.2.2.1	Caregiver role strain
3.2.2.2	High risk for caregiver role strain
3.2.3.1	Parental role conflict
3.3	Altered sexuality patterns

Pattern 4
Valuing: A human response pattern involving the assigning of relative worth

4.1.1	Spiritual distress (distress of the human spirit)

NANDA's *Taxonomy I Revised* — continued

Pattern 5
Choosing: A human response pattern involving the selection of alternatives

5.1.1.1	Ineffective individual coping
5.1.1.1.1	Impaired adjustment
5.1.1.1.2	Defensive coping
5.1.1.1.3	Ineffective denial
5.1.2.1.1	Ineffective family coping: Disabling
5.1.2.1.2	Ineffective family coping: Compromised
5.1.2.2	Family coping: Potential for growth
5.2.1	Ineffective management of therapeutic regimen (individual)
5.2.1.1	Noncompliance (specify)
5.3.1.1	Decisional conflict (specify)
5.4	Health-seeking behaviors

Pattern 6
Moving: A human response pattern involving activity

6.1.1.1.	Impaired physical mobility
6.1.1.1.1	High risk for peripheral neurovascular dysfunction
6.1.1.2	Activity intolerance
6.1.1.2.1	Fatigue
6.1.1.3	High risk for activity intolerance
6.2.1	Sleep pattern disturbance
6.3.1.1	Diversional activity deficit
6.4.1.1	Impaired home maintenance management
6.4.2	Altered health maintenance
6.5.1	Feeding self-care deficit
6.5.1.1	Impaired swallowing
6.5.1.2	Ineffective breastfeeding
6.5.1.2.1	Interrupted breastfeeding
6.5.1.3	Effective breastfeeding
6.5.1.4	Ineffective infant feeding pattern
6.5.2	Bathing or hygiene self-care deficit
6.5.3	Dressing or grooming self-care deficit
6.5.4	Toileting self-care deficit
6.6	Altered growth and development
6.7	Relocation stress syndrome

Pattern 7
Perceiving: A human response pattern involving the reception of information

7.1.1	Body image disturbance
7.1.2	Self-esteem disturbance
7.1.2.1	Chronic low self-esteem
7.1.2.2	Situational low self-esteem
7.1.3	Personal identity disturbance
7.2	Sensory or perceptual alterations (specify — visual, auditory, kinesthetic, gustatory, tactile, olfactory)
7.2.1.1	Unilateral neglect
7.3.1	Hopelessness
7.3.2	Powerlessness

Pattern 8
Knowing: A human response pattern involving the meaning associated with information

8.1.1	Knowledge deficit (specify)
8.3	Altered thought processes

Pattern 9
Feeling: A human response pattern involving the subjective awareness of information

9.1.1	Pain
9.1.1.1	Chronic pain
9.2.1.1	Dysfunctional grieving
9.2.1.2	Anticipatory grieving
9.2.2	High risk for violence: Self-directed or directed at others
9.2.2.1	High risk for self-mutilation
9.2.3	Post-trauma response
9.2.3.1	Rape-trauma syndrome
9.2.3.1.1	Rape-trauma syndrome: Compound reaction
9.2.3.1.2	Rape-trauma syndrome: Silent reaction
9.3.1	Anxiety
9.3.2	Fear

NANDA taxonomy: The ICD translation

NANDA has translated the NANDA taxonomy into a version compatible with the format used by the World Health Organization's *International Classification of Diseases*. Note that the coding in this version is simpler than the coding used in NANDA's *Taxonomy I Revised*.

Choosing		**Y25**	**Altered Physical Regulation**
Y00	**Impaired Family Coping**		
Y00.0	Compromised	Y25.0	Dysreflexia
Y00.1	Disabled	Y25.1	Hyperthermia
Y01	**Health-Seeking Behaviors**	Y25.2	Hypothermia
Y01.0-9	Health-Seeking Behaviors (Specify)	Y25.3	Risk for Infection
		Y25.4	Impaired Thermoregulation
Y02	**Impaired Individual Coping**	**Y26**	**Altered Respiration**
Y02.0	Impaired Adjustment	Y26.0	Impaired Airway Clearance
Y02.1	Decisional Conflict	Y26.1	Impaired Breathing Pattern
Y02.2	Defensive Coping	Y26.2	Impaired Gas Exchange
Y02.3	Impaired Denial	**Y27**	**Altered Tissue Integrity**
Y02.4	Noncompliance	Y27.0	Impaired Oral Mucous Membrane
		Y27.1	Impaired Skin Integrity
Communicating		Y27.2	Risk for Impaired Skin Integrity
Y10	**Impaired Communication**	**Y28**	**Altered Tissue Perfusion**
Y10.0	Verbal	Y28.0	Cardiopulmonary
		Y28.1	Cerebral
Exchanging		Y28.2	Gastrointestinal
Y20	**Altered Bowel Elimination**	Y28.3	Peripheral
Y20.0	Bowel Incontinence	Y28.4	Renal
Y20.1	Colonic Constipation	**Y29**	**Altered Urinary Elimination**
Y20.2	Perceived Constipation		
Y20.3	Diarrhea	Y29.0	Functional Incontinence
Y21	**Altered Cardiac Output**	Y29.1	Reflex Incontinence
Y22	**Altered Fluid Volume**	Y29.2	Stress Incontinence
Y22.0	Deficit	Y29.3	Urge Incontinence
Y22.1	Risk for Deficit	Y29.4	Total Incontinence
Y22.2	Excess	Y29.5	Retention
Y23	**Risk For Injury**		
Y23.0	Aspiration		
Y23.1	Disuse Syndrome		
Y23.2	Poisoning		
Y23.3	Suffocation		
Y23.4	Trauma		
Y24	**Altered Nutrition**		
Y24.0	Less Than Body Requirement		
Y24.1	More Than Body Requirement		
Y24.2	Risk for More Than Body Requirement		

NANDA taxonomy: The ICD translation – *continued*

Feeling

Y30	**Anxiety**
Y31	**Altered Comfort**
Y31.0	Pain
Y31.1	Chronic Pain
Y32	**Fear**
Y33	**Grieving**
Y33.0	Anticipatory
Y33.1	Dysfunctional
Y34	**Post-Trauma Response**
Y34.0	Rape-Trauma Syndrome
Y34.1	Rape-Trauma Syndrome: Compound Reaction
Y34.2	Rape-Trauma Syndrome: Silent Reaction
Y35	**Risk for Violence**

Knowing

Y40	**Knowledge Deficit**
Y40.0-9	Knowledge Deficit (Specify)
Y41	**Altered Thought Processes**

Moving

Y50	**Altered Activity**
Y50.0	Activity Intolerance
Y50.1	Risk for Activity Intolerance
Y50.2	Diversional Activity Deficit
Y50.3	Fatigue
Y50.4	Impaired Physical Mobility
Y50.5	Sleep Pattern Disturbance
Y51	**Bathing or Hygiene Deficit**
Y52	**Dressing or Grooming Deficit**
Y53	**Feeding Deficit**
Y53.0	Impaired Breastfeeding
Y53.1	Impaired Swallowing
Y54	**Altered Growth and Development**
Y55	**Altered Health Maintenance**
Y56	**Impaired Home Maintenance Management**
Y57	**Toileting Deficit**

Perceiving

Y60	**Altered Meaningfulness**
Y60.0	Hopelessness
Y60.1	Powerlessness
Y61	**Altered Self-Concept**
Y61.0	Body Image Disturbance
Y61.1	Personal Identity Disturbance
Y61.2	Self-Esteem Disturbance: Chronic Low
Y61.3	Self-Esteem Disturbance: Situational
Y62	**Altered Sensory Perception**
Y62.0	Auditory
Y62.1	Gustatory
Y62.2	Kinesthetic
Y62.3	Olfactory
Y62.4	Tactile
Y62.5	Visual
Y62.6	Unilateral Neglect

Relating

Y70	**Altered Family Processes**
Y71	**Altered Role Performance**
Y71.0	Parental Role Conflict
Y71.1	Altered Parenting
Y71.2	Risk for Altered Parenting
Y71.3	Sexual Dysfunction
Y72	**Altered Sexuality Patterns**
Y73	**Altered Socialization**
Y73.0	Impaired Social Interaction
Y73.1	Social Isolation

Valuing

Y80	**Altered Spiritual State**
Y80.0	Spiritual Distress

practice data base and international standards for nursing care. Eventually, nurses might be able to obtain separate reimbursement for their services from third-party payers, such as health insurance companies, Medicare, and Medicaid. When this happens, nurses will need billing codes that fit the formats of these payers.

FORMULATING A NURSING DIAGNOSIS
To formulate your nursing diagnoses, you must evaluate the essential assessment information. The following questions will help you quickly zero in on the appropriate data:
• What are the patient's signs and symptoms?
• Which assessment findings are abnormal for this patient?
• How do particular behaviors affect the patient's well-being?
• Which strengths or weaknesses does the patient have that affect his health status?
• Does he understand his illness and treatment?
• How does the patient's environment affect his health?
• How does the patient respond to his health problem? Does he want to change his state of health?
• What kind of relationship does the patient have with his family? What kind of relationships does he have with other members of the community?
• Can the patient problems I've identified be treated with nursing interventions?
• Do I need to gather any further information for my diagnoses?

Selecting a diagnosis from the NANDA list
Becoming familiar with the NANDA taxonomy will help you to formulate nursing diagnoses efficiently and accurately. (See *Tips for using nursing diagnosis terminology.*)

Many nurses complain that the language used in the NANDA taxonomy is confusing. Understanding the syntax of nursing diagnoses can help reduce this confusion. A nursing diagnosis usually consists of a label (a concise term or phrase) with a qualifier.

The diagnostic label describes a health concept. The following are examples of diagnostic labels:
• parenting
• airway clearance
• health maintenance
• swallowing
• social interaction.

Tips for using nursing diagnosis terminology

Developing a working knowledge of the approved nursing diagnoses and their uses will enable you to make the best use of the NANDA list. Here are some tips for improving your familiarity with diagnosis terminology.
• Use a nursing diagnosis manual that provides an up-to-date list of approved diagnoses. You may also refer to the *Quick reference to nursing diagnoses* on pages 236 to 259. New diagnoses are added to the NANDA taxonomy every 2 years after the biennial conference on the classification of nursing diagnoses.
• Study the approved diagnoses that you're most likely to use frequently. Make sure that the reference you use explains each diagnosis and its defining characteristics and provides examples of how to use the diagnosis properly.
• Try to use diagnoses that are understood and accepted by your colleagues. If nurses in your institution disagree about the clinical validity of certain diagnoses, avoid using those diagnoses.
• Practice using nursing diagnoses. Ask your peers or other knowledgeable nurses to provide feedback on your selection of diagnoses.

In these examples, the label is neutral; it has neither positive nor negative connotations until you add a qualifier.

The qualifier is an adjective that clarifies the meaning of the diagnostic label. Examples of NANDA qualifiers include *altered, chronic, decreased, disturbed, dysfunctional, increased, impaired,* and *ineffective.* (See *NANDA-approved qualifiers,* page 68.) Together, the label and qualifier describe a patient problem. Consider the following examples:
• altered parenting
• ineffective airway clearance
• altered health maintenance
• impaired swallowing
• impaired social interaction.

Types of nursing diagnoses
Each nursing diagnosis can be grouped into one of three broad conceptual categories: actual nursing diagnoses, high-risk nursing diagnoses, and wellness nursing diagnoses.

Actual nursing diagnoses describe the patient's current responses to health problems or life processes. They are supported by defining characteristics—deviations from normal that confirm the diagnosis.

High-risk nursing diagnoses describe unhealthful responses that *may* develop in a vulnerable patient. For example,

NANDA-approved qualifiers

This table provides an alphabetized list of qualifiers recommended by NANDA for use in nursing diagnoses. Studying this list will help you to become familiar with nursing diagnosis terminology. In some cases, you may not be able to find a NANDA-approved diagnosis that describes your patient's needs accurately. In such cases, consider using this list to develop your own nursing diagnosis.

QUALIFIER	DEFINITION	QUALIFIER	DEFINITION
Acute	• Severe but of short duration	Dysfunctional	• Abnormal • Incomplete functioning
Altered	• A change from baseline	Excessive	• Amount or quantity greater than necessary, desirable, or useful
Chronic	• Long lasting • Habitual • Constant	Increased	• Greater in size, amount, or degree
Decreased	• Reduced size, amount, or degree	Impaired	• Made worse, weakened • Damaged, reduced • Deteriorated
Deficient	• Inadequate in amount, quality, or degree • Defective • Insufficient • Incomplete	Ineffective	• Not producing the desired effect
Depleted	• Emptied wholly or partially • Exhausted	Intermittent	• Stopping and starting at intervals • Periodic • Cyclic
Disturbed	• Agitated • Interrupted • Experiencing upheaval or interference	Potential for enhanced	• Opportunity to make greater or increase in quality (for use with wellness diagnoses)

suppose you believe that a bedridden patient is in danger of developing pressure ulcers. To document your concerns, you would write *high risk for impaired skin integrity* in your plan of care. High-risk diagnoses are confirmed by the presence of risk factors — environmental, physiologic, psychological, genetic, or chemical — that contribute to the patient's increased vulnerability to an unhealthful event.

Wellness nursing diagnoses describe the potential for the patient to achieve a better state of health. Wellness diagnoses listed in the **NANDA** taxonomy include *health-seeking behaviors, family coping: potential for growth,* and *effective breast-*

feeding. These diagnoses can be formulated using the qualifier *potential for enhanced*—for example, *potential for enhanced family coping, potential for enhanced self-care,* and *potential for enhanced self-esteem.* Wellness diagnoses are especially useful when working in community health settings that focus on promoting health, such as well-baby clinics and schools.

Specialty diagnoses

Some diagnoses in the NANDA taxonomy are geared to specialized practice settings or health problems. For example, *unilateral neglect* occurs when a patient loses perceptual awareness of one side of the body. This state usually occurs in patients with neurologic deficits, such as those who have had a cerebrovascular accident. Another example is *anticipatory grieving,* which occurs when a patient responds to a potential loss. This diagnostic label is especially useful when working with oncology patients and the terminally ill. *Effective breastfeeding* is a wellness diagnosis used in maternity nursing.

Specialty diagnoses are worth learning if you expect to use them. When becoming familiar with nursing diagnoses, concentrate on those that will be most useful to your practice.

Identifying etiologic factors

When formulating a nursing diagnosis, you'll usually want to include a statement identifying etiologic factors. Also known as related factors, etiologic factors are conditions or circumstances that contribute to the development or continuation of the diagnosis. Etiologic factors may include environmental, physiologic, psychological, sociocultural, or spiritual circumstances identified during your analysis of patient assessment data.

Formulating an etiologic statement

When documenting etiologic factors, use the phrase "related to" (or, for short, "R/T") to show that the diagnosis and the etiology have a relationship, though not necessarily a direct cause-and-effect relationship. Examples of nursing diagnoses and related etiologies include the following:
• impaired home maintenance management *related to inadequate support system*
• diversional activity deficit *related to long-term hospitalization*
• hypothermia *related to inadequate clothing*
• sensory or perceptual alteration (visual) *related to insufficient environmental stimuli.*

A single diagnosis may have several possible etiologies. For example, the nursing diagnosis *sexual dysfunction* may be related to any of the following etiologies:
• biological or psychosocial factors
• ineffectual or absent role models
• physical abuse
• psychosocial abuse (harmful relationships)
• vulnerability
• value conflict
• lack of privacy
• altered body structure or function
• lack of knowledge.

Including an etiologic statement will help guide your selection of nursing interventions. The statement should describe phenomena that are amenable to nursing interventions; addressing conditions identified in the etiology should help in selecting interventions to resolve the patient's problem. Keep in mind that the etiologic statement should not be a repetition of the medical diagnosis. Seek to identify etiologic factors during your analysis of patient assessment data.

Writing an accurate etiologic statement takes knowledge and skill. In its publication *Taxonomy I Revised*, NANDA includes suggested etiologies for many nursing diagnoses. Referring to a nursing diagnosis manual may also be helpful; you may want to compare your patient data with etiologic statements included in such references. Also see the nursing diagnosis case studies, pages 77 to 95, for examples of how to formulate a nursing diagnosis with an etiologic statement. Try to be as precise as possible, especially because the etiology largely determines the nursing interventions you'll include in your plan of care.

If you don't know the etiology, write the diagnosis like this: *fatigue related to unknown etiology.* Sometimes, your diagnosis will not require an etiology. For example, the nursing diagnosis *rape-trauma syndrome* does not require an etiology because it is implied in the diagnostic label.

Nursing diagnosis errors

Three kinds of problems can lead to errors in identifying the nursing diagnosis. The problems are:
• *Inaccurate collection of data.* This problem may be the result of poor communication between you and the patient during assessment. The patient may not have understood medical terminology, or he may have given you what he thought were the

proper answers to your questions. Noise, lack of privacy, and other factors also may interfere with your assessment.

• *Inaccurate interpretation of data.* You may begin interpreting data before you've completed your assessment, thus placing too much emphasis on your early impressions. You may jump to conclusions; for example, you may too quickly assign a nursing diagnosis based on the patient's medical diagnosis. Or you may simply make mistakes or succumb to personal biases.

• *Lack of knowledge or experience.* If you don't know about certain problems or have never had experience with them, you'll be less likely to interpret the data correctly. This is a common error for student nurses or nurses who change specialties.

Here are some pointers to help you better analyze patient data:

• Keep an open mind and be aware of your biases.

• Explore alternate possible explanations for the data.

• Develop several possible diagnoses and check to see which fits the data best. Compare associated defining characteristics or risk factors with the patient's signs and symptoms.

• Study the health problems likely to occur in the patient population you work with. Read nursing journals, especially those that describe clinical problems and their relationship to nursing diagnoses.

• Ask the patient what he thinks his problem is. This is called patient verification of the diagnosis.

• Talk with other nurses who are good diagnosticians, and find out how they analyze patient data.

Along with errors in diagnostic reasoning, you may make errors when writing the nursing diagnosis statement. (See *Avoiding errors when writing nursing diagnoses,* pages 72 and 73.) Writing the statement accurately is important because the diagnosis is the basis for selecting patient outcomes, and you are accountable for selecting appropriate interventions and achieving these outcomes. Remember that a nursing diagnosis is the identified response to a health problem or life process.

Writing your own nursing diagnoses

You should make every effort to use diagnoses already approved by NANDA. This helps to create a standard language for communication with colleagues and contributes to the development of an accurate data base to document nursing care and resource use.

However, the NANDA taxonomy is not yet complete. In some cases, you may not be able to find a NANDA-approved

Avoiding errors when writing nursing diagnoses

The following pointers will help you identify and correct common errors made when writing nursing diagnoses.

Don't identify a problem that nursing interventions can't treat. Focus on problems that you can manage through nursing care.

Error
Below-the-knee amputation related to diabetes mellitus

Correction
High risk for impaired skin integrity related to lack of knowledge about stump care and prosthesis management

Don't state a nursing intervention instead of a nursing diagnosis. Revise your statement to describe the patient's response to a health problem or life process.

Error
Intermittent urinary catheterization related to incontinence

Correction
Reflex incontinence related to neuromuscular impairment

Don't describe an appropriate emotional response as unhealthful. Instead, focus on related problems that could interfere with the patient's ability to cope.

Error
Anger related to diagnosis of diabetes

Correction
Noncompliance related to anger about need to follow diabetic diet

Don't let your own biases and value judgments override the patient's perception of his health problems and needs. Diagnoses based on subjective data should be validated by the patient.

Error
Social isolation related to not wanting to see anyone

Correction
No diagnosis may be needed; for example, the patient may prefer to be alone during his illness.

Don't write a legally inadvisable statement.

Error
Ineffective airway clearance related to difficulty with suctioning equipment

Correction
Ineffective airway clearance related to thick, tenacious secretions

Avoiding errors when writing nursing diagnoses — *continued*

Don't write a tautological statement (one in which the label and etiology say the same thing). Revise the etiology to reflect environmental, physiologic, social, psychological, or spiritual factors that contribute to the development or continuation of the diagnosis.

Error	Correction
Sleep pattern disturbance related to frequent awakenings	Sleep pattern disturbance related to unfamiliar surroundings and abdominal pain

Don't reverse the two parts of the statement.

Error	Correction
Lack of understanding of diabetic diet related to noncompliance	Noncompliance related to lack of understanding of diabetic diet

Don't identify a nursing problem instead of a patient problem.

Error	Correction
Difficulty suctioning related to thick secretions	Ineffective airway clearance related to thick tracheal secretions

diagnosis that describes your patient's health problems and needs adequately. When this problem arises, consider devising your own nursing diagnoses. Following NANDA guidelines will help to ensure that your diagnostic statement is accurate.

Preparation
When preparing to write your own nursing diagnosis, cluster objective and subjective data from your assessment of the patient's condition. These data should provide the basis for your choice of terms to label your diagnosis.

Determining the diagnostic concept
Determine which of the three types of nursing diagnoses will best meet your patient's needs: an actual diagnosis, a high-risk diagnosis, or a wellness diagnosis. Keep in mind the following NANDA specifications:
• Actual diagnoses must include a label, an etiology, and defining characteristics.
• High-risk diagnoses must include a label and risk factors.
• Wellness diagnoses must include a label.

Naming the label and qualifier

Start with a label to name the new diagnosis. The label should be a concise term or phrase that represents a pattern or cluster of signs and symptoms or clinical cues — subjective and objective data that prompt you to suspect a health problem.

You may choose to include an appropriate qualifier. You can use one of NANDA's qualifiers: *acute, altered, chronic, decreased, deficient, depleted, disturbed, dysfunctional, excessive, increased, impaired, ineffective, intermittent,* and *potential for enhanced.* Alternatively, you may develop a new qualifier that better meets your patient's needs.

Formulating the etiologic statement

According to NANDA specifications, when writing an actual nursing diagnosis, you must include an etiologic statement. High-risk and wellness diagnoses do not require etiologies. Remember to use "related to" to indicate the relationship between diagnosis and etiology. And keep in mind that a single diagnostic concept can be related to a variety of etiologies.

Formulating the definition

Next, define the new diagnosis. The *definition* should clearly and precisely communicate the meaning of the diagnosis. It should help to differentiate the new diagnosis from similar diagnoses.

Identifying defining characteristics or risk factors

If you're creating an actual diagnosis, the next step is to identify *defining characteristics.* Defining characteristics are clinical findings that, when grouped together, confirm the diagnosis. They may take the form of a list of signs and symptoms or clinical cues. Documenting this information makes it easier for colleagues to understand and use your diagnosis. If you would like to submit your diagnosis to NANDA for approval, documenting defining characteristics is a necessity. Keep the following NANDA criteria in mind:

• A defining characteristic that must be present for the diagnosis to be made is a "critical indicator."

• A defining characteristic that's present 80% to 100% of the time is a "major indicator."

• A defining characteristic that provides supporting evidence for the diagnosis 50% to 79% of the time is considered a "minor indicator."

If you're creating a high-risk nursing diagnosis, you must include *risk factors*. These are environmental, physiologic, psychological, genetic, or chemical factors that increase the patient's vulnerability to the health problem under consideration. Wellness nursing diagnoses do not require defining characteristics or risk factors.

Critiquing your work
Before finishing, you'll want to review your new diagnosis. Check to make sure that the diagnosis does not contain errors. Also make sure that you have not renamed a medical diagnosis. Finally, check to make sure that the NANDA taxonomy doesn't already include an appropriate diagnosis. Look closely at the defining characteristics of diagnoses similar to yours, and compare them with your patient's signs and symptoms.

Submitting your diagnosis to NANDA
If you develop a diagnosis that applies to a large number of patients, consider submitting the diagnosis and your supporting explanation to NANDA. Because the taxonomy is still being developed, NANDA continues to oversee the approval of new nursing diagnoses. (See *The birth of a nursing diagnosis,* page 76.)

You must provide NANDA with the following information: the type of diagnostic concept (actual, high-risk, or wellness), components of the proposed diagnosis (label and qualifier, etiology, definition, and defining characteristics or risk factors, as appropriate), and a sample diagnostic statement.

You should also provide a literature review of the existing body of knowledge concerning the diagnostic concept. This may include research articles; relevant clinical data and descriptions; and references for each defining characteristic, etiology, and risk factor. Your literature review may also include a research validation study conducted on the diagnostic concept. This information may be drawn from case studies, nursing consensus studies, retrospective chart reviews, and other forms of nursing research.

Along with all other material, you should include patient outcome criteria and nurse-prescribed interventions.

For formal guidelines for submitting a diagnosis, write NANDA at 3525 Caroline Street, St. Louis, MO 63104, or call (314) 577-8954.

The birth of a nursing diagnosis

Proposals for new diagnoses come from nursing staff, nurse-educators, nurse-researchers, and student nurses. To be included in the NANDA taxonomy, new diagnoses must undergo a rigorous review process.

Diagnosis Review Committee
Once NANDA receives a proposal for a new diagnosis, information is forwarded to the Diagnosis Review Committee. The committee chair reviews the proposal for completeness and returns it to the author for more information, if necessary. The author has an opportunity to resubmit the proposal. The committee then meets, reviews the proposal, and makes one of three decisions.

The committee may not accept the proposal for further review if:
• the diagnostic concept is a medical diagnosis, a treatment, or a procedure
• the diagnostic concept is not a human response
• the defining characteristics of actual diagnoses are not cues or signs and symptoms
• the defining characteristics of high-risk diagnoses are not risk factors.

Alternatively, the proposal may be held for revisions and returned to the author with a new deadline. Reasons for revisions vary but usually include inadequate literature support or conclusions that go beyond the research presented.

Finally, the Diagnosis Review Committee may decide to accept the proposal.

Expert advisory panel
If the proposal is accepted, it will next be reviewed by an expert advisory panel. The panel may recommend that the proposal be returned to the author for further development (the author may resubmit the proposal for the next review cycle) or that it be accepted conditionally (pending revisions); or the panel may not require any further revisions and may recommend that the diagnosis be included in the taxonomy. The proposal is then forwarded to the NANDA Board of Directors for approval.

Membership vote
The last steps of the approval process take place during and after the national conferences on the classification of nursing diagnoses. These conferences are held once every 2 years. The authors of board-approved nursing diagnoses present their work at the conference. After the conference, NANDA members vote on new diagnoses by mail. A majority of "yes" votes means that the diagnosis will be approved by NANDA for clinical testing, further development, and inclusion in the taxonomy.

NURSING DIAGNOSIS CASE STUDIES

Each of the following case studies describes how to apply a nursing diagnosis in clinical practice.

Activity intolerance

Activity is a basic need—participating in activity creates a sense of autonomy, well-being, and mastery and contributes to physical fitness.

Any factor that interferes with the patient's physical ability, functional status, or energy level may contribute to activity intolerance. The patient who experiences activity intolerance has insufficient physiologic or psychological energy to perform daily activities.

Activity intolerance affects all aspects of the patient's life—physical, psychological, social, cultural, and spiritual. It may lead to overwhelming fatigue, depression, powerlessness, and loss of purpose.

Assessing for activity intolerance
To assess for activity intolerance, evaluate the patient's response to activity. Check for dyspnea, excessive increase in respiratory rate, and an irregular breathing pattern. Also look for bradycardia, tachycardia, arrhythmias, decreased pulse strength, and an excessive increase in blood pressure. The patient may report fatigue or weakness before, during, or after activity. Other signs and symptoms may include:
• avoidance of, lack of interest in, or decreased activity
• decreased muscle tone
• pallor, cyanosis, excessive redness, coolness, or dryness with strenuous activity
• drooped posture.

Activity intolerance may be related to any of the following etiologic factors:
• bed rest
• immobility
• generalized weakness
• sedentary life-style.

Case study
Beth Carson, RN, works in a cardiac care unit. Beth knows that after a major cardiac event, many patients experience decreased cardiac output, which decreases delivery of oxygenated blood to tissues and may lead to activity intolerance.

Alison Pritchert is a 52-year-old lawyer recently admitted with a myocardial infarction (MI). Her hemodynamic status has stabilized and all pressure monitoring has been discontinued. When Beth tells Ms. Pritchert that she'll be getting up to walk around her room later in the day, Ms. Pritchert says, "Oh, I couldn't do that. I'm too tired and still very short of breath. Just moving in my bed wears me out."

That afternoon, when Ms. Pritchert does get up to walk, her pulse becomes irregular and drops to 68 beats/minute, her respirations are 30 breaths/minute and ragged, and her blood pressure remains unchanged. She complains of difficulty breathing and looks pale. She returns to her bed but still feels tired and weak 10 minutes later.

Developing a plan of care

When considering Ms. Pritchert's assessment data, Beth thinks about possible diagnoses: activity intolerance, decreased cardiac output, ineffective individual coping, depression, and fatigue. Although these diagnoses are common in post-MI patients, Beth does not have sufficient assessment data to support all of them.

In light of Ms. Pritchert's remarks and her physiologic response to walking, Beth makes the following diagnosis: *activity intolerance related to an imbalance between oxygen supply and demand.* To support her diagnosis, Beth notes Ms. Pritchert's vital signs after her afternoon walk and documents her remarks and her recovery pattern after activity.

Beth performs a more thorough assessment of Ms. Pritchert's activity pattern before planning activity and rest periods. She needs to know Ms. Pritchert's activity pattern and response before the MI and while in the cardiac care unit. Beth also assesses the significance of activity for Ms. Pritchert—does she associate activity with being able to work, enjoying recreation, being independent, or feeling exhausted? When writing her plan of care, Beth includes the following nursing interventions:
• *Encourage adequate rest periods before walking, meals, and diagnostic procedures.* Beth will have to help Ms. Pritchert develop a rest schedule that does not exacerbate activity intolerance. She'll also need to communicate this schedule to the health care team.
• *Teach Ms. Pritchert to monitor her activity level and take a rest when she becomes fatigued.* This not only promotes independence but also prepares Ms. Pritchert for monitoring her own activity after discharge. Learning to monitor activity may also help her cope with the fear of having another MI.
• *Discuss the importance of increasing activity tolerance.* Teaching is aimed at helping Ms. Pritchert understand how exercise contributes to cardiac risk factor reduction.
• *Help Ms. Pritchert progress in the cardiac exercise program as her tolerance increases.* This is a standard program for all cardiac patients.

Developing expected outcomes

Based on the nursing diagnosis of activity intolerance, Beth includes the following expected outcomes in Ms. Pritchert's plan of care:
• Vital signs remain within normal limits during and after activity.
• Patient plans appropriate activity and rest periods.
• Patient participates in the cardiac exercise program.

Summary

• Activity intolerance occurs when the patient has insufficient energy to complete daily activities.
• Assessment for activity intolerance should include monitoring physiologic responses to activity and listening for comments about fatigue or weakness.

• Patients who have a condition that affects oxygen supply or who have been on prolonged bed rest are at risk for activity intolerance.
• Nursing interventions for treating this diagnosis include performing an in-depth assessment of responses to activity, planning rest and activity periods, teaching about the need for activity, and implementing an activity program.

Altered health maintenance

Any patient who cannot identify or manage health problems or fails to seek help to maintain his health may experience altered health maintenance. For the patient with a chronic illness, this nursing diagnosis is a major concern. Such a patient must have basic knowledge and skills to maintain his health as well as specific knowledge and skills to manage the disease and its treatment.

Poor health maintenance may result in physical complications, debilitation, ineffective coping, depression, and other problems. One of the major functions of patient education and discharge planning is to prevent this diagnosis.

Assessing for altered health maintenance
The major defining characteristics of this diagnosis are lack of knowledge about basic health practices or needed treatments and poor adaptation to internal or environmental changes. Other defining characteristics include:
• inability to take responsibility for basic health practices
• impaired or absent personal support system
• history of poor health-seeking behaviors
• verbalized interest in improving health behaviors
• lack of equipment, finances, or other needed resources.

To detect altered health maintenance, observe your patient or ask him questions about how he manages his health or treatment regimen. Does he know about healthy living habits? If he has a chronic illness, does he follow his medication regimen correctly? Does he monitor his responses to the disease and seek help when appropriate? Does he make choices that support or jeopardize his health?

Case study
Jenny Chu, RN, works in an endocrine clinic in the Midwest, helping diabetic patients implement their treatment regimens. Many of her patients have psychosocial problems that make the demands of coping with diabetes more complex. For some patients, adhering to the medical regimen may interfere with social life. Other patients may not want to follow recommendations made by health professionals. Additional problems that interfere with health maintenance may include:
• lack of communication skills
• lack of personal autonomy
• ineffective individual coping
• ineffective family coping
• inadequate time and energy
• inaccessibility of information and services
• complete or partial lack of gross or fine motor skills.

Viola Smith, age 38, has had insulin-dependent diabetes mellitus for 23 years. She is beginning to develop diabetic complications and recently has been experiencing three or more episodes of hypoglycemia per week. Jenny's colleagues report that Mrs. Smith is a difficult patient who complains frequently and does not follow recommendations.

When Jenny enters the examining room, Mrs. Smith briefly looks up but never establishes eye contact. Mrs. Smith is 5"6" and weighs 350 lb; her blood pressure is 145/95 mm Hg and her vital signs are within normal limits. Her hair is oily but she appears to be clean. She complains of fatigue, nausea, and diarrhea.

Mrs. Smith tells Jenny that she does not monitor her blood sugar but tries to follow her diet. However, her husband, who does the family shopping, likes fried foods, and she fixes and eats whatever he buys. Mrs. Smith adds, "It's too difficult for me to shop. I get tired walking around the store, plus I live in a second floor apartment and I just can't manage the stairs very well."

Jenny then asks Mrs. Smith what she does for recreation. "My best time is watching the daytime talk shows. My husband buys me this really good chocolate. I feel good when I eat it. I have chocolate every day while watching Phil or Oprah."

Then Mrs. Smith describes her insulin routine. "I do it just the way the doctor said. I take it right after I get up in the morning and then right before dinner."

Because Mrs. Smith has so many hypoglycemic attacks, Jenny asks her to describe her routine more precisely. Mrs. Smith explains her schedule: wake up with husband at 7 a.m., take insulin, get him off to work, return to bed, wake up around 10 a.m., have lunch about 11 a.m., watch TV, clean a little, husband returns home, take insulin, eat dinner, watch TV, and go to bed about 11 p.m. Mrs. Smith does not eat breakfast.

Developing a plan of care

When considering Mrs. Smith's assessment data, Jenny lists possible diagnoses: altered health maintenance, ineffective individual coping, noncompliance, body image disturbance, knowledge deficit, and social isolation. Although each of these diagnoses may apply to Mrs. Smith, Jenny does not have the assessment data to support all of them.

Jenny considers Mrs. Smith's daily routine, her desires and needs, and her knowledge of the diabetic regimen. She makes the following nursing diagnosis: *altered health maintenance related to lack of knowledge and lack of adaptive behaviors.* This diagnosis is based upon Mrs. Smith's description of her daily routine, her insulin regimen and food pattern, her lack of knowledge about glucose monitoring, and her lack of exercise and frequent consumption of chocolate.

Jenny believes that nursing care should be geared toward helping Mrs. Smith develop a daily pattern that promotes health and yet fits in with her life-style and beliefs. To foster a sense of empowerment, she realizes that she must enlist Mrs. Smith's participation in designing this new daily pattern. Jenny develops the following nursing interventions:

• *Help Mrs. Smith establish personal health goals, including an achievable diet plan and exercise program.* Jenny makes an appointment with Mrs. Smith to begin working on mutual goal setting. Since Mrs. Smith's main complaint is fatigue, Jenny discusses how lack of exercise, a high-fat diet, and uncontrolled blood glucose levels may contribute to fatigue. She asks Mrs. Smith to keep a log monitoring fatigue, which they will use to start setting achievable personal health goals.

• *Teach glucose monitoring skills.* Jenny decides to postpone this intervention until Mrs. Smith's next visit so that she can check various monitoring options. Along with teaching how and when to monitor blood glucose levels, Jenny will design a person-alized insulin dosage and administration schedule for Mrs. Smith.

• *Develop an insulin management plan.* For now, Jenny sticks with Mrs. Smith's origi-nal insulin orders. However, she emphasizes that Mrs. Smith must eat immediately after taking her insulin, not 3 or 4 hours later. Then Jenny talks about the need to establish a plan that will encourage Mrs. Smith to assume responsibility for insulin management.

• *Teach about hypoglycemia.* Jenny does this quickly with a handout because the clinic visit is almost over. She emphasizes Mrs. Smith's individual responses to hypo-glycemia and how to manage them. Jenny makes a note to review this material at Mrs. Smith's next visit and to ask follow-up questions about hypoglycemic episodes.

• *Assess available resources to assist with activities of daily living.* Mrs. Smith has rea-sons for not doing many things for herself. Jenny needs more information before she can determine if Mrs. Smith will benefit from support services.

Developing expected outcomes
Based on the nursing diagnosis of altered health maintenance, Jenny includes the fol-lowing expected outcomes in Mrs. Smith's plan of care:
• Patient achieves mutually developed health goals.
• Patient keeps a record of insulin and glucose values.
• Patient takes insulin at appropriate times.
• Patient experiences less than one episode of hypoglycemia per week.
• Patient seeks and uses available resources to assist with activities of daily living.

Summary
• Altered health maintenance occurs when a patient cannot identify or manage health problems or fails to seek help to maintain health.
• When assessing for altered health maintenance, look for evidence of lack of knowl-edge about basic and therapeutic health practices and poor ability to adapt to inter-nal or environmental changes.
• Patients with chronic illnesses are at high risk for altered health maintenance.
• Nursing interventions to treat altered health maintenance include patient teaching, assessing motivation and health beliefs, mutually agreeing on behavior changes, and encouraging the patient to use available support resources.

Dysreflexia

A patient who's had a spinal cord injury at or above T7 for 3 months or more is at risk for dysreflexia (also known as autonomic dysreflexia). Dysreflexia is a life-threat-ening, uninhibited sympathetic response of the nervous system to a noxious stimu-lus. Factors that place spinal cord injury patients at high risk for dysreflexia include:

• bladder distention
• bowel distention
• skin irritation (abrasions, burns, pressure ulcers)
• menstrual cramps or uterine contractions
• severe pain
• disease processes with visceral symptoms.

A lifelong problem for spinal cord injury patients, dysreflexia is best treated by eliminating the noxious stimulus.

Assessing for dysreflexia

Dysreflexia occurs abruptly; the patient experiences a sense of urgency and a feeling that something is very wrong. Blood pressure rises suddenly (above 140/90 mm Hg). The patient becomes diaphoretic above the injury, develops red splotches on the skin above the injury site and pallor below it, develops bradycardia or tachycardia (less than 60 or more than 100 beats/minute), and complains of a headache.

Other signs and symptoms of dysreflexia include:
• chills
• conjunctival congestion
• Horner's syndrome (contraction of the pupil, partial ptosis of the eyelid, and absence of facial sweating)
• paresthesia
• pilomotor reflex (gooseflesh)
• blurred vision
• chest pain
• metallic taste in mouth
• nasal congestion.

Case study

Julio Ortiz, RN, works in a regional spinal cord injury rehabilitation center. Julio knows that to help his patients live successfully with spinal cord injury, he must teach them the possibilities, limitations, and dangers associated with their condition. He also knows that his patients must learn to prevent dysreflexia and to treat it if it occurs.

Kyle Matthews is a 19-year-old man with a C6-C7 spinal cord lesion caused by a car accident. During a physical therapy session, he suddenly becomes diaphoretic with red splotchy skin above C7 and pale skin below C7. His pulse rate is 140 beats/minute, and his blood pressure is 170/120 mm Hg. He keeps saying, "Something bad is happening, something real bad. I don't feel good. My head hurts real bad."

The physical therapist pages Julio. He arrives within minutes, assesses Kyle, and immediately begins treatment for dysreflexia. Emergency interventions include:
• placing Kyle in a sitting position (the patient's head must be elevated to more than 45 degrees)
• instituting seizure precautions
• looking for and eliminating the source of noxious stimuli (Julio discovers that Kyle's indwelling urinary catheter is kinked and that his bladder is distended; he adjusts the catheter to reestablish urine flow)
• monitoring vital signs every 3 to 5 minutes while looking for the cause, then until vital signs return to baseline
• notifying the doctor and administering any prescribed medications.

After returning Kyle to his room, Julio documents the event in Kyle's chart. Later, Julio talks with Kyle about the experience. Kyle is fearful and says that nothing like that ever happened to him before. He wonders if it will happen again and whether he can handle it by himself.

Developing a plan of care

When reviewing his plan of care, Julio thinks about the event and Kyle's reaction and comments. He forms the following nursing diagnosis: *high risk for dysreflexia related to lack of knowledge and possible bladder distention.* To support his diagnosis, Julio notes that Kyle is having difficulty learning to manage his indwelling urinary catheter (even though he does well at bowel training and pressure ulcer prevention) and does not assume responsibility for checking the tubing during various activities throughout the day.

Julio begins to develop a plan of care to help Kyle learn to prevent or manage dysreflexia. This plan must also include Kyle's primary caregiver, since Kyle will never be completely independent. Julio includes the following nursing interventions in his plan of care:

• *Teach Kyle and his caregiver about the causes and treatment of dysreflexia.* Julio sets up a meeting with Kyle and his primary caregiver, his mother, to begin talking about dysreflexia. He introduces Kyle and his mother to other patients who've experienced dysreflexia and managed it successfully. He supplements these sessions with films, literature, and demonstrations on how to handle the problem if it occurs.

• *Teach prevention strategies.* Julio uses discussion and literature to teach Kyle and his mother ways to prevent dysreflexia. He stresses watching for any noxious stimuli that may cause a nervous system response. He explains that the stimulus could be as minor as accidentally hitting Kyle's foot on his wheelchair. Tight clothing or tight-fitting appliances could also be to blame.

• *Monitor Kyle's bowel and bladder program and his skin breakdown prevention program.* Because bowel and bladder distention and pressure ulcers are prime sources of noxious stimuli, Julio wants to keep track of Kyle's bowel, bladder, and skin care programs. Preventing a recurrence of dysreflexia may require modifying Kyle's regimen.

Developing expected outcomes

Based on the nursing diagnosis of high risk for dysreflexia, Julio includes the following expected outcomes in his plan of care:

• Patient and caregiver state causative factors, signs and symptoms, and interventions for dysreflexia.

• Patient and caregiver implement strategies to prevent dysreflexia.

Summary

• Patients with spinal cord injuries at or above T7 are at risk for dysreflexia, a life-threatening, uninhibited sympathetic response of the nervous system to a noxious stimulus, such as a full bladder or bowel. Dysreflexia can be treated by elevating the patient's head and removing the noxious stimulus.

• Preventing recurrence of dysreflexia may require instituting programs to monitor and eliminate noxious stimuli.

• Patient and caregiver education is essential in preventing and treating dysreflexia.

Health-seeking behaviors

One of the first wellness diagnoses to be accepted by NANDA, health-seeking behaviors applies to an individual in stable health who actively seeks ways to improve personal health habits or make his environment more healthful. For this diagnosis to be accurate, the patient must enjoy good health or any chronic disease processes must be well controlled. This distinction differentiates health-seeking behaviors from altered health maintenance. This is an important diagnosis for nurses who work in health promotion and disease prevention settings.

Assessing for health-seeking behaviors
To justify a diagnosis of health-seeking behaviors, the patient must request assistance in achieving a higher level of health. Without this request, the diagnosis cannot be made. Other defining characteristics include:
• desire for increased control of health practices
• concern about effect of environmental conditions on health status
• unfamiliarity with wellness community resources
• lack of knowledge about health promotion behaviors.

Case study
Nancy Miller, RN, is a cardiac rehabilitation nurse who works at a community hospital. She conducts a cardiac risk factor evaluation and reduction program as part of her facility's primary prevention services. Because many of the risk factors for cardiac disease result from long-term life-style choices, Nancy is aware that many family members of cardiac patients share similar life-style risk factors.

Mary Frances Wilkins is the 56-year-old wife of Marvin Wilkins, who recently had successful coronary artery bypass surgery. During one of Mr. Wilkins's follow-up visits to the hospital, Mrs. Wilkins asks if she can undergo a health risk evaluation. Her husband had undergone such an evaluation as part of his treatment program.

Mrs. Wilkins returns to the hospital the following week for the evaluation. Nancy tells her that her cholesterol level is fine and notes that Mrs. Wilkins has never smoked, a definite plus. However, Mrs. Wilkins is 30 lb overweight and does not exercise regularly—risk factors that need to be modified.

Mrs. Wilkins agrees that her weight is a problem but states that all the women in her family are "pleasantly plump." She does not agree that lack of exercise is a risk factor; after all, she's active all day long with housework, charity work, grandchildren, and gardening. But she says that she's willing to learn more because she wants to set a good example for her husband.

Developing a plan of care
Nancy considers the risk factor profile results and Mrs. Wilkins's statements about her weight and current exercise activities. She notes that Mrs. Wilkins also lacks knowledge about the importance of aerobic exercise. Nancy makes the diagnosis *health-seeking behaviors* because Mrs. Wilkins is healthy and has requested help in becoming healthier. (Remember, a wellness diagnosis does not have an etiology.)

Nancy realizes that lifelong habits are difficult to change. She must work closely with Mrs. Wilkins to develop a program to modify eating and exercise patterns with which Mrs. Wilkins can be successful. Nancy includes the following interventions in her plan of care:

• *Encourage Mrs. Wilkins to enroll in a weight-control and exercise program.* These programs provide education and support for the health goals in which Mrs. Wilkins indicated interest.

• *Recommend that Mrs. Wilkins attend a values clarification program.* Mrs. Wilkins's ideas about her life-style are at odds with her desire to improve her health status. Before her behavior can change, she may need to clarify or alter her values. The hospital has a values clarification program for this purpose.

• *Promote participation in a support group.* Learning new skills and behaviors can be easier with a support group. Group members can help each other plan strategies and can provide positive feedback. Nancy recommends a support group designed for cardiac patients and spouses to learn about healthy life-styles and to cope with the stresses of living with cardiac disease.

Developing expected outcomes
Based on the nursing diagnosis of health-seeking behaviors, Nancy includes the following expected outcomes in Mrs. Wilkins's plan of care:

• Client adopts a personalized exercise program that includes cardiopulmonary fitness.
• Client achieves ideal weight by a mutually agreed upon date.
• Client participates in a support group.

Summary
• Health-seeking behaviors is a wellness nursing diagnosis for patients in good health who want more information or assistance in achieving higher levels of health. A request for information or assistance is the critical indicator for this diagnosis.

• Family members and friends of patients with a chronic illness frequently request health promotion information.

• Effective nursing interventions for this diagnosis include performing a risk factor profile analysis, providing health education, encouraging participation in a support group, and mutually agreeing on behavior changes.

Ineffective airway clearance

Normally, the upper and lower airways have mechanisms to maintain patency. The upper airway heats, humidifies, and filters foreign matter, enabling a person to sneeze or blow matter from his nose or swallow liquid matter. Defense mechanisms in the lower airway include coughing, macrophage clearance, and mucociliary clearance. Anything that interferes with these mechanisms can obstruct the airways, resulting in ineffective airway clearance. If ineffective airway clearance is not diagnosed or treated promptly, the patient may suffer severe pulmonary complications.

Assessing for ineffective airway clearance
Auscultate the patient's chest using a stethoscope. Listen for abnormal breath sounds, such as crackles and rhonchi, which reveal that secretions are pooling in the lungs and that the patient can't cough them up. Also listen to the patient cough. Is the cough effective at moving secretions? Other possible indications of ineffective airway clearance include:
• changes in rate or depth of respirations
• tachypnea
• cyanosis
• dyspnea.
    Factors that put patients at high risk for ineffective airway clearance include:
• tracheobronchial infection, obstruction, or secretions
• decreased energy
• fatigue
• trauma
• perceptual or cognitive impairment.

Case study
Rachel Rubin, RN, works on a surgical unit in a large university hospital. Most of her patients are over age 50 and have had major surgery. They require aggressive pulmonary care to prevent atelectasis and respiratory infection. Preoperative medications and anesthetics cause large amounts of dry, tenacious secretions to form. Many patients complain of fatigue and pain, which impair their ability to breathe deeply and cough effectively.
    Velma Calkins is a 63-year-old woman recently admitted to the surgical unit after an exploratory laparotomy. During auscultation, Rachel hears bilateral crackles in Mrs. Calkins's lung bases. She asks Mrs. Calkins to cough to assess whether or not Mrs. Calkins can clear the crackles. Her cough is weak and produces no sputum; the crackles remain. Rachel then looks at the intake and output sheet and sees that Mrs. Calkins has not been drinking fluids. Rachel notices that Mrs. Calkins tries to cough again but stops and complains of pain around her incision site. Mrs. Calkins also tells Rachel that sometimes it's hard to breathe deeply and that she feels short of breath.

Developing a plan of care
When developing her plan of care, Rachel thinks about Mrs. Calkins's signs and symptoms. She arrives at a diagnosis of *ineffective airway clearance related to fatigue, pain, and thick tracheobronchial secretions.* To support her diagnosis, Rachel notes Mrs. Calkins's ineffective cough, dyspnea, and bilateral crackles.
    Next, Rachel plans interventions. Her goals are to control Mrs. Calkins's pain, increase fluid intake, and decrease fatigue. She knows from working with elderly surgical patients that Mrs. Calkins will need a lot of encouragement. Nursing interventions include:
• *Provide hydration to liquefy secretions.* Because Mrs. Calkins has no other serious health problems, Rachel orders 2,400 ml of fluids daily, taking note of Mrs. Calkins's fluid preferences (tea, cranberry juice, and cold water with a little bit of lemon).

• *Encourage turning, coughing, and deep breathing at least every 2 hours.* Rachel teaches Mrs. Calkins how to cough more effectively and how to splint her chest to decrease pain.

• *Use an incentive spirometer at least four times per hour.* Rachel teaches Mrs. Calkins how to use the spirometer correctly and monitors spirometer use periodically.

• *Auscultate the lungs every 4 hours and as needed.* This enables Rachel to monitor the effectiveness of treatment.

• *Administer analgesics about 30 minutes before ambulation and sessions of deep breathing.* Properly timed medication administration may prevent pain from interfering with deep breathing and coughing and from depressing respirations.

• *Have the patient ambulate as soon as possible.* Prolonged bed rest may contribute to retained secretions, ineffective breathing patterns, and fatigue.

Developing expected outcomes
Based on the nursing diagnosis of ineffective airway clearance, Rachel includes the following expected outcomes in Mrs. Calkins's plan of care:

• Patient's lungs are clear on auscultation.

• Patient states that she can breathe deeply and that her cough effectively clears secretions.

Summary
• Ineffective airway clearance occurs when an obstruction of the airway interferes with normal ventilation.

• Ineffective airway clearance may result from decreased energy or fatigue; trauma; tracheobronchial infection, obstruction, or secretions; or perceptual or cognitive impairment that impairs the ability to notice or manage secretions.

• Assessment for ineffective airway clearance should include auscultating the lungs and evaluating the patient's cough.

• Ineffective airway clearance is common in patients who undergo surgery and experience fatigue, pain, or prolonged bed rest.

• Nursing interventions for ineffective airway clearance include helping the patient breathe deeply and cough, controlling factors that interfere with coughing, keeping secretions loose and thin so that they can be removed easily, and encouraging the patient to walk or at least be as active as possible while on bed rest.

Pain

Pain refers to a subjective state during which an individual experiences and reports discomfort. Unmanaged pain can be a devastating experience — suffering can be extreme and can have major psychological consequences. Pain may interfere with addressing other nursing and medical diagnoses.

Coordinating the management of acute pain is an important nursing responsibility. Your goal is to increase patient comfort and promote conservation of energy.

Assessing for pain
The patient's report of pain is the most important assessment information. Other signs and symptoms include:
• physiologic responses – blood pressure, pulse rate, and respiratory rate changes; dilated pupils; diaphoresis; increased muscle tension
• facial mask of pain – the "beaten" look
• moaning, crying, whimpering, rubbing, pacing
• impaired thought processes
• protective or guarding behavior
• restlessness, agitation, irritability.

Case study
Steve Kline, RN, works on the surgical floor of a university hospital. The most common problem he manages is acute postoperative pain. When documenting this nursing diagnosis for his patient, the most common etiology he writes is "related to the surgical experience."

Steve considers himself an expert in pain relief: He knows appropriate dosages per body weight for the various pain-killing drugs and equianalgesic dosages for narcotic drugs. Steve also uses nonpharmacologic pain-relief measures. He feels that it's his responsibility to provide the best possible pain management for his patients.

Stella Romanowski, age 43, had a cholecystectomy 2 days ago. This is her second day to walk, but the first day to take a walk out of her room. When Steve comes in to walk with her, Mrs. Romanowski says, "I hurt too much. My stomach feels like it's falling out. I just can't do anything. Turn out the light and leave me alone."

Steve asks her how much pain she has. Mrs. Romanowski tells him, "It's horrible." He then assesses her incision and vital signs. The incision looks good, but the vital signs are elevated. Mrs. Romanowski's face is drawn and she has assumed a position that protects her incision. Steve checks her chart. Her last pain medication was given over 5 hours ago and Mrs. Romanowski has not requested another pill. She says she hates to be a bother and complain so much, and besides, it wasn't this bad an hour ago. Steve asks her what she does at home when she has pain. "I just take some aspirin and go to bed," she explains. Steve medicates her and lets her rest.

Developing a plan of care
Mrs. Romanowski has said she's in pain, so Steve adds that diagnosis to the plan of care. He then begins to consider the etiology of the diagnosis. The surgery is an obvious cause, but there are other related factors. He enters the diagnosis *pain related to the surgical experience and lack of knowledge of pain-control techniques.* To support his diagnosis, he notes Mrs. Romanowski's usual pain-control methods, the fact that she had not requested medication, and her vital signs.

Steve then begins to plan strategies that Mrs. Romanowski might use to control her pain. Realizing that it would be too much to ask a patient in pain to participate in planning, he decides to offer Mrs. Romanowski a variety of pain-control options. He documents the following nursing interventions in his plan of care:

• *Assess the pain on a scale of 1 to 10, with 10 being the worst possible pain.* This will help the nursing staff evaluate the efficacy of the pain-control methods.
• *Medicate Mrs. Romanowski 30 minutes before any activity.* Activity periods should be coordinated with rest periods and medication administration.
• *Teach Mrs. Romanowski when and how to request pain medications.* This will give her permission to request medication and promote a sense of control.
• *Teach Mrs. Romanowski several nonpharmacologic strategies to control pain.* Steve feels that Mrs. Romanowski might benefit from deep-breathing techniques, muscle relaxation exercises (but not those that cause muscle tensing, which would increase pain), visualization, and distraction, using her favorite TV shows and movie videos.

Developing expected outcomes
Based on the nursing diagnosis of pain, Steve includes the following expected outcomes in Mrs. Romanowski's plan of care:
• Patient reports feelings of pain to nursing staff.
• Patient implements measures to reduce or eliminate pain.
• Patient is pain-free without medication by discharge.

Summary
• The nursing diagnosis of pain refers to the patient's experience of discomfort.
• A verbal report of pain is the critical indicator for this diagnosis.
• Unmanaged pain can be a devastating experience—suffering can be extreme and can have major psychological consequences.
• Nursing interventions to treat pain include administering prescribed medications and teaching the patient distraction, visualization, and relaxation techniques.

Powerlessness

Any patient who receives care is forced to sacrifice a certain degree of control over his life. Once he enters the health care system, the patient becomes increasingly dependent on others and is expected to defer to the expertise of health care professionals. Disease and hospital confinement circumscribe his mobility. Recovery is largely beyond his control. Further, the patient may not be given enough information to fully understand his illness and its treatment. All these factors may contribute to the patient's feelings of powerlessness.

Powerlessness may become debilitating if the patient stops believing that his own actions have any meaning or influence at all. The patient may become depressed; feelings of hopelessness may prevent him from setting goals and from taking action to achieve his full potential.

Assessing for powerlessness
How can you assess for this nursing diagnosis? Perhaps the best way is by listening to your patient. He may directly express his feeling that he has lost control over his life. Listen for general statements indicating apathy, such as "I don't care." The patient may express hopelessness when physical deterioration continues despite adher-

ence to the health care regimen. He may express frustration over his inability to perform activities of daily living. Other possible indications of powerlessness include:
• diminished interest in self-care
• general discomfort or anxiety
• passivity
• periodic displays of irritability, resentment, anger, or guilt
• expressions of inadequacy and self-doubt.

Case study
June Pinder, RN, works in a nursing home in the Midwest. Most of her patients are over age 80. June recognizes that her patients need more than physiologic care; they need help contending with isolation, boredom, and diminished self-worth. Many have lost spouses, homes, and friends. Further, elderly nursing home patients are at an especially high risk for powerlessness because of the following factors:
• loss of sensory and motor function
• restrictions placed on residents in a long-term care facility
• inability to fulfill their usual social, vocational, and family roles.

Fanny Brightman is an 83-year-old woman recently admitted to the nursing home where June works. During her initial assessment interview, Mrs. Brightman told June that it was not her choice to enter the nursing home. "That decision was made by my children," she said.

Mrs. Brightman's health history assessment revealed that she has had arthritis for the past 15 years and that her ability to take care of herself was rapidly diminishing. Her children felt that they could not take care of her and decided a nursing home would be best.

During her first few days at the nursing home, Mrs. Brightman was withdrawn. She took little interest in the other residents and did not participate in any of the activities available to nursing home residents. Staff members assumed that her behavior was a reflection of her personality. June, however, felt that her withdrawn behavior might be a response to her recent loss of independence and the decline in her level of functioning.

About a week after Mrs. Brightman's admission, June entered her room to perform a preliminary range-of-motion assessment. During the assessment, Mrs. Brightman made several statements about feeling helpless. She blamed her mental state on her declining physical condition and on the limitations imposed by living in a nursing home. She made repeated complaints about her new life-style, such as "It's like living in a prison. No one lets you do anything."

Developing a plan of care
When reviewing her plan of care, June reconsiders Mrs. Brightman's remarks and adds the nursing diagnosis *powerlessness related to loss of control over motor function and living conditions*. To support her diagnosis, June notes Mrs. Brightman's expressions of helplessness, withdrawn behavior, and comments about living in a nursing home.

June's next challenge is to develop a strategy to help minimize Mrs. Brightman's feelings of powerlessness. As a patient advocate, June believes it is her responsibility to empower the nursing home residents in every way possible. She knows from her working experience that fostering the right of the elderly patient to be included in the decision-making process is an important first step.

Her nursing interventions include:
• *Work with Mrs. Brightman on identifying aspects of life that are still under her control.* June arranges a conference to discuss scheduling of daily activities, meals, and physical therapy sessions with Mrs. Brightman. She emphasizes that Mrs. Brightman, not the staff, has the authority to make these decisions. She also mentions that Mrs. Brightman can request changes in the arrangement of furniture in her room if she wishes. June feels that emphasizing Mrs. Brightman's right to make decisions will help prevent powerlessness from becoming overwhelming, especially during the first weeks of Mrs. Brightman's stay at the nursing home.
• *Make colleagues aware of Mrs. Brightman's special needs.* June decides to take steps to ensure that staff nurses who carry out the plan of care will be sensitive to Mrs. Brightman's need to overcome powerlessness. In the plan of care, she directs the nursing staff to allow Mrs. Brightman the opportunity to express her feelings and to set aside time to listen attentively. She further advises her colleagues to express interest in Mrs. Brightman's progress in the physical therapy program.

Developing expected outcomes
Based on the nursing diagnosis of powerlessness, June includes the following expected outcomes in Mrs. Brightman's plan of care:
• Patient expresses positive feelings about her abilities, her living conditions, and herself.
• Patient participates in physical therapy program and in social and recreational activities of her choosing.
• Patient participates in decisions about her own care and life-style.

Summary
• Powerlessness occurs when the patient stops believing that his own actions have any meaning or influence on the outcome of events.
• Listening to the patient is the best way to assess for this diagnosis. Often the patient will make statements that indicate he feels he has lost control over his life.
• Elderly patients in long-term care facilities are especially prone to powerlessness.
• Powerlessness can be effectively treated through nursing action. Important nursing interventions include allowing the patient to express his feelings, listening attentively to the patient, pointing out the aspects of life where the patient still has control, and encouraging the patient to take an active role in health care and life-style decisions.

Social isolation

Social isolation occurs when a patient does not have sufficient contact with his usual support systems. Understanding how the patient perceives his solitude is key to formulating this nursing diagnosis. The patient experiencing social isolation believes that his loneliness has been imposed by others. He perceives aloneness to be negative and threatening. Social isolation may lead to feelings of rejection, low self-worth, depression, loneliness, and hopelessness.

Any patient admitted to the hospital may experience a degree of social isolation. Separated from loved ones, the patient may feel that others are ignoring him as a result of the stigma of his illness. When a patient requires isolation precautions, the risk for social isolation increases.

Social isolation may have adverse health effects. Research shows that the level of social support a patient receives can influence his recovery.

Assessing for social isolation

Because it is a subjective nursing diagnosis, social isolation must be confirmed by statements made by the patient. Listen for comments indicating that the patient feels lonely or rejected by others. Other possible signs and symptoms include:
• uncommunicative, withdrawn affect
• poor eye contact
• expression of feeling different from others
• expression of frustration over inability to meet others' expectations
• expression of lack of purpose in life
• preoccupation with own thoughts
• projection of hostility in voice and behavior
• seeking to be alone.

Social isolation may be related to any of the following etiologic factors:
• unacceptable social behavior
• inadequate support systems
• inability to engage in satisfying personal relationships
• impaired mobility
• alteration in mental status
• alteration in physical appearance.

Case study

Cindy Farr, RN, works on a bone marrow transplant unit, where many patients are placed in reverse isolation. She knows her patients are at high risk for the nursing diagnosis of social isolation. Visitors are few and limited in number. Some family members and friends don't even visit because they're afraid of "catching cancer."

Joel McAndrew is a 17-year-old who has recently had a bone marrow transplant and is now in reverse isolation. Although his room is filled with cards and gifts from friends and family, only his mother visits regularly. His father and two brothers visit occasionally. Joel used to call his friends frequently, but he has stopped in the last few days. He says he just doesn't have anything in common with them any more. At times he expresses anger at his family for not visiting more often. He tells Cindy, "They have their own lives and don't care about me any more. So they don't come. Who needs them?" Joel no longer enjoys his hobbies: listening to music, reading science fiction novels, and watching music videos.

When Cindy tries to involve Joel in activities, he becomes angry and tells her to "get lost." He says he doesn't need anyone any more. His appetite has begun to diminish.

Developing a plan of care

As Cindy considers Joel's assessment data, she thinks about possible diagnoses: social isolation, impaired social interaction, altered thought processes, self-esteem disturbance, and ineffective individual coping. Although each of these diagnoses may apply to Joel, Cindy does not have assessment data to support all of them. Cindy considers Joel's statements about his friends and family, his hostility, and his decreased involvement with favorite activities. She makes the following nursing diagnosis: *social isolation related to reverse isolation and inability to engage in satisfying personal relationships.* To support her diagnosis, Cindy notes Joel's lack of social support as well as his comments.

Cindy has to decide how to address this nursing diagnosis. Part of the solution, she believes, is to encourage friends and family to visit more frequently. But because social isolation is a subjective state, even a substantial increase in visits might not make Joel feel less isolated. She and Joel need to have a long talk about his feelings. Cindy writes the following nursing interventions in her plan of care:

• *Spend time with Joel during each shift.* This gives Joel an opportunity to talk about his sense of isolation. By listening to him, Cindy can communicate concern and encourage Joel to initiate interaction with others.

• *Encourage Joel to use the telephone to communicate more with friends and family.* He should also consider sending cards and letters.

• *Find out why other family members don't visit.* Cindy can't assume that all family members are afraid of cancer or are disinterested. Other barriers may make it difficult for family members to visit.

• *Encourage visits from Joel's friends.* Friends may not be aware of how important their visits are, or they may be afraid of making Joel sicker because he is in reverse isolation.

• *Set limits on Joel's hostile behavior.* His behavior could drive more people away from him, thus increasing his isolation.

• *Obtain a consultation for diversional therapy.* This may help Joel to focus on activities rather than on his solitude.

Developing expected outcomes

Based on the nursing diagnosis of social isolation, Cindy includes the following expected outcomes in Joel's plan of care:
• Patient talks about his social isolation.
• Patient contacts family and friends.
• Patient maintains control over expression of angry feelings.

Summary

• Social isolation occurs when a patient experiences a sense of aloneness that he considers to be imposed by others.
• Listening for statements about feeling alone or nobody caring is critical in assessing for social isolation.
• Any hospitalized patient is vulnerable to social isolation; patients in isolation have an especially high risk of developing this nursing diagnosis.

• Nursing interventions for social isolation include setting limits on undesirable behavior, arranging for contact with social support systems, and helping the patient to talk about his feelings of isolation.

Stress incontinence

The patient with stress incontinence experiences small amounts of urine loss (50 ml or less) with abdominal pressure. A distressing and socially disruptive condition, stress incontinence occurs most commonly among postmenopausal women and among young women after childbirth. Mild stress incontinence can usually be treated with nursing interventions. More complex problems may require medical interventions.

Assessing for stress incontinence
To overcome patient embarrassment, you'll need to ask open-ended questions and establish a trusting relationship during assessment. Initially, the patient may complain of leaking urine. Take a voiding history to determine the circumstances that precipitate incontinence as well as the frequency and timing of the episodes. With the patient in lithotomy, sitting, and standing positions, observe the urinary meatus for dribbling.

Signs and symptoms of stress incontinence may include:
• urinary urgency
• urinary frequency
• small-volume urine loss
• little or no nocturia
• leakage with exercise, coughing, laughing, or lifting.

Stress incontinence may be related to any of the following etiologic factors:
• excessive weight
• multiple pregnancies
• weak pelvic muscles
• traumatic childbirth
• estrogen deficiency
• weak sphincter tone
• history of pelvic surgeries
• overdistention between voidings.

Case study
Sylvia DeMarco, RN, works in a women's clinic. Women come to the clinic for health screening, common gynecologic problems, and postpartum follow-up care. Sylvia has developed expertise in managing urinary tract problems.

Susan Jamison is a 27-year-old mother of four young children. Throughout her pregnancies, she has gained a lot of weight. Before beginning a strenuous weight-loss program, she must undergo a Papanicolaou test and a check-up. She is 5'6" and weighs 200 lb.

During the physical examination, Mrs. Jamison mentions that she's worried about her weight-loss exercise program because whenever she moves too much, she leaks a small amount of urine. When she goes out for the day, she wears a pad. She knows incontinence is common for elderly women but is a little distressed that it is happening to her at so young an age. She confides that "sometimes it's very embarrassing."

Sylvia examines Mrs. Jamison for the extent of stress incontinence. With Mrs. Jamison in the lithotomy position, Sylvia asks her to cough and detects no leakage. Next, Mrs. Jamison sits upright and coughs; a few drops of urine leak out. Finally, Mrs. Jamison stands up and coughs; she passes about 30 ml of urine. Sylvia finds that Mrs. Jamison has very weak pelvic muscle tone.

Developing a plan of care

Based on the assessment data, Sylvia adds the following nursing diagnosis to Mrs. Jamison's plan of care: *stress incontinence related to obesity and weakened pelvic floor muscles*. To support her diagnosis, Sylvia notes a history of multiple pregnancies, obesity, and results of the physical examination.

Sylvia then begins planning Mrs. Jamison's care. Because the plan will require lifestyle changes, Sylvia will have to work very closely with Mrs. Jamison. Sylvia feels that with patients like Mrs. Jamison, she can best serve as coach and support person. Sylvia includes the following interventions in her plan of care:

• *Teach Kegel exercises.* These exercises are designed to strengthen pelvic floor muscles so that they can resist the pressure of urine in the bladder. It takes about 6 months for results to become apparent.

• *Teach abdominal muscle exercises.* Typically, supporting structures of the bladder and urethra are weak.

• *Plan a weight-loss program.* Obesity is a major contributor to increased abdominal pressure, which stimulates urine leakage. Sylvia will need to encourage Mrs. Jamison to adhere to her diet.

• *Plan an exercise program that avoids jarring exercise.* Jarring exercise can increase episodes of urine leakage.

• *Have Mrs. Jamison keep a voiding record.* Mrs. Jamison should empty her bladder about every 2 hours to decrease the chance of leakage. Maintaining a record will help ensure accurate evaluation of care.

Developing expected outcomes

Based on the nursing diagnosis of stress incontinence, Sylvia includes the following expected outcomes in Mrs. Jamison's plan of care:

• Patient maintains optimal dryness at all times.

• Patient achieves continence in 6 months.

Summary

• Stress incontinence involves urine loss of 50 ml or less and is associated with increased abdominal pressure. Verbal reports of urine leakage and direct observation can confirm the diagnosis.

• Women who are obese, who've had multiple pregnancies, or who are postmenopausal are at risk for stress incontinence.

• Stress incontinence can be treated with muscle-strengthening exercises and reduction of other risk factors. In some cases, medical care may be needed.

KEY POINTS

• A nursing diagnosis is a clinical judgment about a patient's response to health problems or life processes. Nursing diagnoses provide the basis for the selection of nursing interventions. You are accountable for achieving patient outcomes associated with each nursing diagnosis.

• Even though medical and nursing diagnoses sometimes overlap, you should be aware of important differences between the two. Your nursing diagnoses describe the patient problems that your nursing interventions can help resolve. Some of these problems may occur secondary to medical treatment. If you plan your care of a patient around only the medical aspects of his illness, you'll probably overlook significant problems.

• The North American Nursing Diagnosis Association (NANDA) has developed the most widely accepted standardized list of nursing diagnoses — the NANDA taxonomy.

• The NANDA taxonomy categorizes nursing diagnoses according to nine human response patterns: exchanging, communicating, relating, valuing, choosing, moving, perceiving, knowing, and feeling.

• Each nursing diagnosis can be grouped into one of three broad conceptual categories: actual diagnoses, high-risk diagnoses, and wellness diagnoses.

• Actual nursing diagnoses are confirmed by defining characteristics — clinical findings that indicate an unhealthful human response. High-risk diagnoses are confirmed by risk factors — environmental, physiologic, psychological, genetic, or chemical — that contribute to the patient's increased vulnerability to an unhealthful event.

• The nursing diagnosis statement begins with a label — a concise term or phrase that describes a health concept. The label may be modified by a qualifier — an adjective chosen to clarify the diagnostic label.

• When formulating a nursing diagnostic statement, you'll usually want to include a statement identifying etiologic factors. Also known as related factors, etiologic factors are conditions or circumstances that contribute to the development or continuation of the diagnosis.

• The etiologic statement should describe conditions that are amenable to nursing interventions; it should not be a repetition of the medical diagnosis.

• Because the NANDA taxonomy is not complete, you may not be able to find a NANDA-approved diagnosis that describes your patient's needs adequately. When this problem arises, consider devising your own nursing diagnoses.

1. A nursing diagnosis is:

   a. a translation of a medical diagnosis into the domain of nursing.

   b. a phrase or term describing a patient care task performed by a nurse.

   c. a clinical judgment about human responses to health problems or life processes.

   d. an evaluation of a patient's medical needs made by a nurse in an emergency situation.

   e. all of the above.

2. How does a nursing diagnosis differ from a medical diagnosis?

   a. A nursing diagnosis may change as the patient's responses change.

   b. A nursing diagnosis may apply to the patient's family as well as to the patient himself.

   c. A nursing diagnosis focuses on the patient's perception of his health status as well as on his physical condition.

   d. Formulating a nursing diagnosis is within the legally permissible scope of nursing practice.

   e. All of the above.

3. The NANDA taxonomy:

   a. organizes nursing diagnoses under categories called human response patterns.

   b. arranges medical diagnoses so that they can be incorporated into the nursing plan of care.

   c. lists nursing diagnoses according to Maslow's hierarchy of needs.

   d. provides a systematic method for keeping track of tasks to be accomplished for each patient.

   e. none of the above.

4. Which one of the following is *not* a human response pattern?

    a. moving
    b. choosing
    c. relating
    d. valuing
    e. sharing

5. Which one of the following most accurately describes the components that should be included when developing a nursing diagnosis?

    a. diagnostic label with qualifier
    b. diagnostic label with qualifier and defining characteristics
    c. diagnostic label with qualifier, defining characteristics, and assessment data
    d. diagnostic label with qualifier, defining characteristics, and etiology
    e. diagnostic label with qualifier, etiology, and risk factors

6. Name the error in this diagnostic statement: Pain related to myocardial infarction.

    a. There is no error; the statement is written correctly.
    b. The statement reflects an inappropriate value judgment.
    c. Both parts of the statement (label and etiology) say the same thing.
    d. The etiology is a medical diagnosis.
    e. The statement is legally inadvisable.

7. Name the error in this diagnostic statement: Impaired home maintenance management related to laziness and lack of effort.

    a. There is no error; the statement is written correctly.
    b. The diagnostic label describes a patient problem that is not within the domain of nursing.
    c. The statement reflects an inappropriate value judgment.
    d. Both parts of the statement (label and etiology) say the same thing.
    e. The diagnosis identifies an appropriate emotional response as unhealthful.

8. Name the error in this diagnostic statement: Ineffective individual coping related to lack of social support.

   a. There is no error; the statement is correct as written.
   b. The diagnostic label identifies an appropriate emotional response as unhealthful.
   c. The statement is legally inadvisable.
   d. The statement reflects an inappropriate value judgment.
   e. The statement identifies a nursing problem instead of a patient problem.

9. Name the error in this diagnostic statement: Anger related to death of spouse.

   a. There is no error; the statement is written correctly.
   b. The diagnostic label identifies an appropriate emotional response as unhealthful.
   c. Both parts of the statement say the same thing.
   d. The etiology is a medical diagnosis.
   e. The statement indicates a cultural bias.

10. Name the error in this diagnostic statement: Daily tracheostomy care related to mucus buildup.

   a. There is no error; the statement is written correctly.
   b. The diagnostic label identifies a nursing treatment instead of a patient problem.
   c. Nursing interventions can't treat the problem. The etiology is a medical diagnosis.
   d. The two parts of the statement (label and etiology) are reversed.
   e. The statement is legally inadvisable.

(For answers with rationales, turn to page 261.)

FURTHER READINGS

Abdellah, F.G. *Patient Centered Approach to Nursing.* New York: Macmillan Publishing Co., 1960.

Bulechek, G.M., and McCloskey, J.C. *Nursing Interventions: Essential Nursing Treatments,* 2nd ed. Philadelphia: W.B. Saunders Co., 1992.

Carroll-Johnson, R.M., ed. *Classification of Nursing Diagnoses: Proceedings of the Eighth Conference.* Philadelphia: J.B. Lippincott Co., 1989.

Carroll-Johnson, R.M., ed. *Classification of Nursing Diagnoses: Proceedings of the Ninth Conference.* Philadelphia: J.B. Lippincott Co., 1991.

Carroll-Johnson, R.M., ed. *Classification of Nursing Diagnoses: Proceedings of the Tenth Conference.* In press. Philadelphia: J.B. Lippincott Co.

Fitzpatrick, J.J., et al. "Translating Nursing Diagnosis into ICD Code," *AJN* 89(4):493-95, April 1989.

Gebbie, K.M., ed. *Summary of the Second National Conference: Classification of Nursing Diagnoses.* St. Louis: Clearing-house — National Group for Classification of Nursing Diagnoses, 1976.

Gebbie, K.M., and Lavin, M.A., eds. *Classification of Nursing Diagnoses: Proceedings of the First National Conference.* St. Louis: Mosby-Year Book, Inc., 1975.

Gebbie, K.M., and Lavin, M.A. "Classifying Nursing Diagnoses," *AJN* 74(2):250-53, February 1974.

Gordon, M. *Manual of Nursing Diagnosis, 1991-1992.* St. Louis: Mosby-Year Book, Inc., 1991.

Gordon, M. *Nursing Diagnosis: Process and Application,* 2nd ed. New York: McGraw-Hill Book Co., 1987.

Hannah, K.J., et al., eds. *Clinical Judgement and Decision Making: The Future with Nursing Diagnosis (Proceedings of the International Conference).* Albany, N.Y.: Delmar Pubs., Inc., 1987.

Hurley, M.E., ed. *Classification of Nursing Diagnoses: Proceedings of the Sixth Conference.* St. Louis: Mosby-Year Book, Inc., 1986.

Kim, M.J., and Moritz, D.A., eds. *Classification of Nursing Diagnoses: Proceedings of the Third and Fourth National Conferences.* New York: McGraw-Hill Book Co., 1982.

Kim, M.J., et al., eds. *Classification of Nursing Diagnoses: Proceedings of the Fifth National Conference.* St. Louis: Mosby-Year Book, Inc., 1984.

McLane, A.M., ed. *Classification of Nursing Diagnoses: Proceedings of the NANDA Conference, 7th.* St. Louis: Mosby-Year Book, Inc., 1987.

McManus, R.L. *Assumptions of the Functions of Nursing.* New York: Columbia University, 1950.

Monograph of the Invitational Conference on Research Methods for Validating Nursing Diagnoses. St. Louis: North American Nursing Diagnosis Association, 1989.

Mundinger, M., and Jauron, G. "Developing a Nursing Diagnosis," *Nursing Outlook* 23(2):94-98, February 1975.

Nursing: A Social Policy Statement. Kansas City, Mo.: American Nurses' Association, 1980.

Sparks, S.M., and Taylor, C.M. *Nursing Diagnosis Reference Manual,* 2nd ed. Springhouse, Pa.: Springhouse Corp., 1993.

Standards of Nursing Practice. Kansas City, Mo.: American Nurses' Association, 1991.

Taxonomy I Revised. St. Louis, Mo.: North American Nursing Diagnosis Association, 1990.

Warren, J.J. "Accountability and Nursing Diagnosis," *Journal of Nursing Administration* 13(10):34-37, October 1983.

Warren, J.J., and Hoskins, L.M. "The Development of NANDA's Nursing Diagnosis Taxonomy," *Nursing Diagnosis* 1(4):162-68, October-December 1991.

Yura, H., and Walsh, M.B. *The Nursing Process: Assessing, Planning, Implementing, Evaluating,* 5th ed. East Norwalk, Conn.: Appleton & Lange, 1987.

CHAPTER 4

PLANNING

The third step of the nursing process involves creation of a plan of action that will direct your patient's care toward desired goals. Drafted with guidance from your patient and members of the health care team, the plan of care serves as a written record of your patient's nursing diagnoses, expected outcomes, nursing interventions, teaching plan, and evaluation data.

In this chapter, you'll find full information on how to develop an appropriate plan of care, including:
• establishing care priorities
• identifying expected outcomes
• formulating nursing interventions to attain expected outcomes
• documenting the plan in the format required by your facility.

Because nursing care is dynamic, you'll need to review and revise your plan regularly, based on your patient's progress and changes in the treatment regimen.

WHY PREPARE A PLAN OF CARE?
The plan of care provides the health care team with a central source of information about the patient's problems, needs, and goals. It gives direction by showing colleagues the goals established for the patient and by providing instructions to achieve them. It also provides necessary actions for solving patient problems and for dealing with any unexpected complications.

For example, if your plan includes instructions on ambulation, this information can be used by other nurses, nursing assistants, and the physical therapist. Providing colleagues with a written plan reduces the risk of misunderstanding, safeguards against duplication of services, and helps ensure continuity of care on all shifts and by staff from other departments.

In an era of diminishing health care resources, maintaining an accurate plan of care is especially important. The soaring cost of health care has increased the emphasis on

Ensuring a successful plan of care

Your plan of care must rest on a solid foundation of carefully chosen nursing diagnoses. It also must fit your patient's needs, age, developmental level, culture, strengths and weaknesses, and willingness and ability to take part in his care. Your plan should help the patient attain the highest functional level while posing minimal risk and without creating new problems. If complete recovery isn't possible, your plan should help the patient cope physically and emotionally with his impaired or declining health.

Using the following guidelines will help ensure that your plan of care is effective:
• Be realistic. Avoid setting a goal that's too difficult for the patient to achieve. The patient may become discouraged, depressed, and apathetic if he can't achieve expected outcomes.
• Tailor your approach to each patient's problem. Individualize both your outcome statements and nursing interventions. Keep in mind that each patient is different; no two patient problems are exactly alike.
• Avoid vague terms; instead, use quantitative, precise terms. For example, if your patient is restless, describe his specific behavior: "picks at bed clothes," "pulls at restraints," or "screams or moans." To indicate that the patient's vital signs are stable, document specific measurements, such as "heart rate less than 100 beats/minute" or "systolic blood pressure greater than 100 mm Hg."

measuring the effectiveness and quality of health care delivery. By documenting accurate, measurable outcome statements, you can substantiate the effectiveness of nursing care and thereby help to justify the allocation of nursing resources. By improving communication and ensuring continuity of treatment, your plan of care can promote increased quality of care (see *Ensuring a successful plan of care*).

SETTING PRIORITIES
Many patients have multiple problems, which in turn require multiple nursing diagnoses. Once you've formulated your patient's nursing diagnoses, you'll need to determine which problems require immediate attention and which can wait.

Always give the highest priority to problems that threaten your patient's life or pose immediate safety risks. Ask yourself: "Will my patient's life be endangered if this problem isn't addressed immediately?" Next, give priority to your patient's nonemergency needs. Lower-priority diagnoses involve needs that don't relate to the patient's specific illness or prognosis.

Suppose, for example, you're caring for a patient with insulin-dependent diabetes mellitus, related problems caused by diabetic retinopathy, and insufficient knowledge of diabetes treatment. You'd give top priority to making sure the patient follows the medical regimen because failure to administer insulin could lead to death. You'd assign second priority to addressing the patient's vision deficit to lessen the risk of injury from falls. Once your patient was physiologically stable and the risk for injury had declined, you could address other nursing needs, such as the need for teaching to encourage compliance.

Keep in mind that addressing the most fundamental problem first may help resolve other problems, either directly or indirectly. And, sometimes, you can address several problems simultaneously. For your insulin-dependent diabetic patient with a leg ulcer, for example, you might decide to address his lack of knowledge about diabetes treatment while caring for his ulcer. Your interventions might include discussing the need to control his diabetes while changing his dressing.

Must the plan of care address all of the patient's problems? No — provided that these problems are routine, such as hygiene, toileting, or dressing. However, when unusual factors or special considerations exist, the patient's needs should be documented in the plan of care.

Maslow's hierarchy of needs
Abraham Maslow described five levels of human needs, arranged hierarchically from the most basic to the most abstract. He proposed that survival needs must be met before higher-level ones (those less crucial to survival) can be addressed. In fact, higher-level needs may not become apparent until lower-level needs are at least partially met (see *Understanding Maslow's hierarchy of needs*).

Maslow's hierarchy is especially useful in establishing priorities for a patient with multiple nursing diagnoses. For example, a victim of abuse may need his physical injuries treated (physiologic needs). Next, he may need protection from the abuser (safety and security) and then support and reassurance (love and belonging). Long-term goals may include helping the patient to establish a sense of self-worth and independence (self-esteem and self-actualization). To understand how nursing diagnoses may be incorporated into Maslow's scheme, see *Arranging nursing diagnoses by Maslow's hierarchy of needs*, pages 106 and 107.

Understanding Maslow's hierarchy of needs

Maslow's hierarchy provides a system for classifying human needs that may prove useful when establishing priorities for your patient's care. Maslow described five levels of human needs, with basic physiologic needs forming the lowest level of the pyramid and self-actualization needs forming the highest.

The diagram below depicts Maslow's hierarchy of needs. Shown at left is the ascending hierarchy of human needs; the definitions at right explain the need categories.

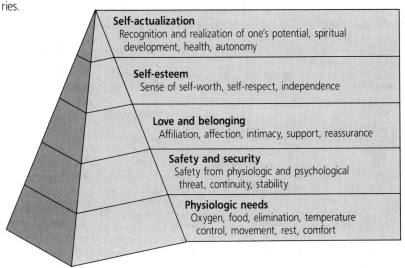

Self-actualization
Recognition and realization of one's potential, spiritual development, health, autonomy

Self-esteem
Sense of self-worth, self-respect, independence

Love and belonging
Affiliation, affection, intimacy, support, reassurance

Safety and security
Safety from physiologic and psychological threat, continuity, stability

Physiologic needs
Oxygen, food, elimination, temperature control, movement, rest, comfort

In 1983, Kalish refined Maslow's hierarchy by subdividing physiologic needs into survival needs and stimulation needs and adding esteem for others to self-esteem needs. The diagram below depicts Kalish's refinement of Maslow's model.

Self-actualization

Esteem for self and others

| Love | Belonging | Closeness |

| Safety | Security | Protection |

| Sex | Activity | Exploration | Manipulation | Novelty |

| Food | Air | Water | Temperature | Elimination | Rest | Pain avoidance |

Arranging nursing diagnoses by Maslow's hierarchy of needs

Maslow's hierarchy of needs stipulates that lower-level physiologic needs must be met before higher-level abstract needs can be met. Considering need categories as you identify patient problems will help you decide which nursing diagnoses to address first. The chart below groups nursing diagnoses according to the categories in Maslow's hierarchy.

Physiologic needs
- Activity intolerance
- Airway clearance, ineffective
- Aspiration, high risk for
- Body temperature, altered, high risk for
- Breast-feeding, effective
- Breast-feeding, ineffective
- Breast-feeding, interrupted
- Breathing pattern, ineffective
- Cardiac output, decreased
- Constipation (colonic, perceived)
- Diarrhea
- Fatigue
- Fluid volume deficit
- Fluid volume excess
- Gas exchange, impaired
- Hyperthermia
- Hypothermia
- Incontinence (bowel, functional, reflex, stress, total, urge)
- Infant feeding pattern, ineffective
- Mobility, impaired
- Nutrition, altered
- Oral mucous membrane, altered
- Pain
- Pain, chronic
- Peripheral neurovascular dysfunction, high risk for
- Protection, altered
- Self-care deficit (specify)
- Sensory or perceptual alteration
- Sexual dysfunction
- Sexuality pattern, altered
- Skin integrity, impaired
- Sleep pattern disturbance
- Swallowing, impaired
- Thermoregulation, ineffective
- Thought processes, altered
- Tissue integrity, impaired
- Tissue perfusion, altered
- Urinary elimination pattern, altered
- Urinary retention
- Ventilation, spontaneous: Inability to sustain
- Ventilatory weaning response, dysfunctional

Safety and security
- Anxiety
- Disuse syndrome, high risk for
- Dysreflexia
- Fear
- Grieving, anticipatory
- Grieving, dysfunctional
- Health maintenance, altered
- Home maintenance management, impaired
- Infection, high risk for
- Injury, high risk for
- Management of therapeutic regimen, ineffective
- Neglect, unilateral
- Poisoning, high risk for
- Self-mutilation, high risk for
- Suffocation, high risk for
- Trauma, high risk for
- Verbal communication, impaired

Love and belonging
- Caregiver role strain
- Caregiver role strain, high risk for
- Coping, family: Potential for growth
- Coping, ineffective family
- Family processes, altered
- Parental role conflict
- Parenting, altered
- Social interaction, impaired
- Social isolation

Arranging nursing diagnoses by Maslow's hierachy of needs – *continued*

Self-esteem
- Adjustment, impaired
- Body image disturbance
- Coping, defensive
- Coping, ineffective family
- Coping, ineffective individual
- Decisional conflict
- Denial
- Diversional activity deficit
- Hopelessness
- Noncompliance
- Personal identity disturbance
- Posttrauma response
- Powerlessness

- Rape-trauma syndrome
- Relocation stress syndrome
- Role performance, altered
- Self-esteem, chronic low
- Self-esteem, situational low
- Self-esteem disturbance
- Violence, high risk for

Self-actualization
- Growth and development, altered
- Health-seeking behaviors
- Knowledge deficit
- Spiritual distress

Keep in mind that self-esteem needs may have to be addressed in any hospitalized patient who must depend on others for meeting his needs.

Richard Kalish expanded Maslow's hierarchy by subdividing the first need level into survival needs and stimulation needs. Survival needs, the lowest level of Kalish's pyramid, include food, air, water, temperature, elimination, rest, and avoidance of pain. When a deficit occurs in any of these areas, the patient will tend to use all available resources to fill that deficit. Stimulation needs, the second level, include sex, activity, exploration, manipulation, and novelty. After meeting survival needs, the patient must address stimulation needs before ascending the hierarchy. For example, a patient on prolonged bed rest may need to participate in self-care and diversionary activities to progress in therapy and achieve greater independence.

Orem's universal self-care demands theory

Dorothea Orem's theory offers an alternative framework for determining patient care priorities. Orem defines self-care as the activities a person performs to maintain life, health, and well-being. To maintain integrated human functions, all individuals must meet universal self-care demands. In this theory, Orem describes the following as universal self-care demands:

• adequate intake of air, water, and food
• adequate elimination of waste
• achieving a balance between activity (mental and physical) and rest
• achieving a balance between solitude and social interaction
• prevention of hazards
• promotion of human functioning (establishing normality and avoiding stress).

If an individual can't satisfactorily meet these demands, the nurse intervenes by providing and managing care. According to Orem's theory, the goals of nursing include helping the patient overcome circumstances that interfere with self-care and cause limitations and deficits.

You can use Orem's framework to help assign care priorities. Under her system, your first priority is to address problems that interfere with the patient's routine physiologic functioning, such as his ability to breathe or maintain adequate circulation. Next, consider the patient's elimination patterns and activity needs. Once these problems have been addressed, you can focus on the effects of illness or injury on the patient's behavior. (See *Arranging nursing diagnoses by Orem's universal self-care demands*.)

Soliciting patient input
Involving your patient in planning is crucial to ensuring successful nursing care. Ideally, you'll set care priorities together with the patient and his family.

Effective communication is essential when working with the patient and family to establish care priorities. The following guidelines may help to improve communication:
• Create a quiet, private, and unhurried environment. Keep all communication factual and direct.
• Encourage the patient and family members to ask questions regarding the plan of care.
• Describe goals and interventions in simple, clear language.
• Ask the patient to summarize the content of his plan of care, and check the accuracy of his response.
• Clarify missing or misunderstood information.

In some cases, you may believe that the patient's choice of priorities will interfere with your ability to administer appropriate care. For example, the patient may want to address a relatively unimportant problem first because he doesn't understand the possible consequences of delaying treatment of a more important problem. In such a case, you may need to pro-

Arranging nursing diagnoses by Orem's universal self-care demands

According to Orem, all individuals must meet *universal self-care demands*. If an individual cannot satisfactorily meet these demands, the nurse intervenes by providing and managing care. Because Orem's theory suggests a progression from basic physiologic needs to higher levels of human functioning, you can use it to set priorities for patient care problems. The following list arranges nursing diagnoses according to Orem's universal self-care demands.

Air
• Airway clearance, ineffective
• Aspiration, high risk for
• Breathing pattern, ineffective
• Gas exchange, impaired
• Ventilation, spontaneous: Inability to sustain
• Ventilatory weaning response, dysfunctional

Water
• Cardiac output, decreased
• Fluid volume deficit
• Fluid volume deficit, high risk for
• Fluid volume excess
• Tissue perfusion, altered

Food
• Breast-feeding, effective
• Breast-feeding, ineffective
• Breast-feeding, interrupted
• Infant feeding pattern, ineffective
• Nutrition, altered: Less than body requirements
• Nutrition, altered: More than body requirements
• Nutrition, altered, high risk for: More than body requirements
• Oral mucous membrane, altered

Elimination
• Constipation
• Constipation, colonic
• Constipation, perceived
• Diarrhea
• Incontinence, bowel

• Incontinence, functional
• Incontinence, reflex
• Incontinence, stress
• Incontinence, total
• Incontinence, urge
• Skin integrity, impaired
• Skin integrity, impaired, high risk for
• Urinary elimination pattern, altered
• Urinary retention

Activity and rest
• Activity intolerance
• Activity intolerance, high risk for
• Disuse syndrome, high risk for
• Diversional activity deficit
• Fatigue
• Mobility, impaired
• Neglect, unilateral
• Self-care deficit
• Sleep pattern disturbance

Solitude and social interaction
• Family processes, altered
• Parental role conflict
• Parenting, altered
• Parenting, altered, high risk for
• Rape-trauma syndrome
• Role performance, altered
• Self-mutilation, high risk for
• Sexual dysfunction
• Sexuality pattern, altered
• Social interaction, impaired
• Social isolation
• Verbal communication, impaired
• Violence, high risk for

(continued)

Arranging nursing diagnoses by Orem's universal self-care demands *– continued*

Prevention of hazards
- Body temperature, altered, high risk for
- Dysreflexia
- Health maintenance, altered
- Health-seeking behaviors
- Home maintenance management, impaired
- Hyperthermia
- Hypothermia
- Infection, high risk for
- Injury, high risk for
- Management of therapeutic regimen, ineffective
- Noncompliance
- Pain
- Pain, chronic
- Peripheral neurovascular dysfunction, high risk for
- Poisoning, high risk for
- Protection, altered
- Suffocation, high risk for
- Swallowing, impaired
- Thermoregulation, ineffective
- Tissue integrity, impaired
- Trauma, high risk for

Promotion of human functioning
- Adjustment, impaired
- Anxiety

- Body image disturbance
- Caregiver role strain
- Caregiver role strain, high risk for
- Coping, defensive
- Coping, family: Potential for growth
- Coping, ineffective family
- Coping, ineffective individual
- Decisional conflict
- Denial
- Fear
- Grieving, anticipatory
- Grieving, dysfunctional
- Growth and development, altered
- Hopelessness
- Knowledge deficit
- Personal identity disturbance
- Posttrauma response
- Powerlessness
- Relocation stress syndrome
- Self-esteem, chronic low
- Self-esteem, situational low
- Self-esteem disturbance
- Sensory or perceptual alteration
- Spiritual distress
- Thought processes, altered

---

vide additional teaching to the patient and encourage him to reexamine the values underlying his choices. You must, however, bear in mind the principle of autonomy – the ethical and legal right of the patient to make his own decisions about health care.

IDENTIFYING EXPECTED OUTCOMES
After setting care priorities, you'll need to identify expected outcomes. Expected outcomes are measurable, patient-focused goals that are derived from the patient's nursing diagnoses. They serve as the basis for evaluating the effectiveness of nursing care. You may find that a single nursing diagnosis may require more than one expected outcome.

An expected outcome can specify an improvement in the patient's ability to function, such as an increase in the distance he can walk. Or it can specify an amelioration of a problem, such as reduction of pain. Each outcome statement should call for the greatest improvement realistically possible for your patient.

Writing the outcome statement

Documenting expected outcomes accurately is crucial to the success of your plan of care. Expected outcome statements that are vague, hard to measure, or unrealistic can invalidate a plan that's otherwise accurate and useful.

An outcome statement should include four components:
• the specific behavior that will show the patient has reached his goal
• criteria for measuring the behavior (specifying how much, how long, how far, and so on)
• conditions under which the behavior should occur
• the target date or time by which the behavior should occur.

Including target dates in your outcome statement is important. Target dates can help motivate your patient, especially when he meets a goal ahead of schedule, and they're crucial for evaluating the quality of your plan of care. Also, realistic target dates can help your health care facility evaluate nursing effectiveness.

When writing an outcome statement, use the following guidelines.

Make your statement specific

Use specific action verbs, such as *walks, demonstrates, drinks, eats,* and *expresses.* A vague statement, such as "Patient improves nutritional intake," provides colleagues sharing the plan with little to go on. Instead, clearly state which behaviors you expect the patient to exhibit and when. A more specific statement would read: "Patient consumes 1,200 calories daily by 3/28/93."

Focus on the patient

Your outcome statement shouldn't describe a nursing action. Instead, describe the desired effects of nursing care on patient behavior. Don't write: "Nurse helps patient walk 10 feet q.i.d." Instead write: "Patient walks 10 feet with help q.i.d."

Encourage patient participation
As with other aspects of planning, involve your patient in developing outcome statements. Besides helping you to set more realistic goals, this will help motivate the patient.

Consider medical orders
Make sure you don't write outcome statements that ignore or contradict medical orders. For example, before writing the outcome statement "Patient walks 10 feet unassisted q.i.d. by 4/4/93," make sure the medical orders don't call for more restricted activity.

Adapt the outcome to the circumstances
Take into account the patient's coping ability, age, educational level, religious and cultural influences, family support, living conditions, and socioeconomic status. When setting target dates for achieving goals, consider his anticipated length of stay. In some cases, you'll need to consider the health care setting itself. For instance, the outcome statement "Patient will walk outdoors with help for 20 minutes t.i.d. by 5/30/93" may be unrealistic in a large city hospital.

Consider revisions
You may need to revise even the most carefully written outcome statement. If your patient has trouble reaching his goal, you may have to revise a target date or change the goal to one he can reach more easily. The trend toward earlier discharge may necessitate more frequent revisions to avert reimbursement problems.

Developing learning outcomes
You may document your patient-teaching plan as part of your plan of care or as a separate plan. Today, many health care facilities require a separate plan because of the emphasis placed on teaching by accrediting and regulatory organizations. The need to control costs and discharge patients earlier further underscores the importance of teaching plans.

A teaching plan identifies what your patient needs to learn, how he'll be taught, and criteria for evaluating how well he learns. Like the expected outcomes you write for patient care, those you write for patient learning must describe measurable and observable behavior and must focus on the patient, not the nurse. Learning outcomes should convey what you're going to teach, the behavior you expect to see, and the criteria for evaluating what the patient has learned.

Start each learning outcome statement with a precise action verb, and limit each to a single task. An appropriate learning outcome for the patient who must give himself injections would be: "Patient demonstrates insulin withdrawal in a syringe by Friday, July 9."

DEVELOPING NURSING INTERVENTIONS
After establishing expected outcomes, you'll develop interventions designed to help the patient achieve these outcomes and write detailed intervention statements to communicate your ideas to other staff members. Follow these guidelines when developing nursing interventions.

Consider the etiologic portion of the diagnostic statement
The related etiology should guide the choice of nursing interventions. For example, if the diagnostic statement reads *hyperthermia related to dehydration*, you'd determine interventions for alleviating the dehydration. Such interventions might include determining the patient's preference for liquids, keeping liquids at bedside, monitoring intake and output, and administering I.V. fluids.

Tailor the intervention to your patient
Consider such factors as your patient's condition, age, developmental and educational levels, environment, and values. The more you know about the patient, the easier it will be to formulate appropriate interventions. For example, if your patient is scheduled for cardiac catheterization and has a reading disability, don't write an intervention for patient teaching that includes sophisticated reading material from the American Heart Association. Instead, try to incorporate a teaching videotape or audiotape into your plan.

Keep the patient's safety in mind
One of your main responsibilities is to maintain a safe environment for your patient. You must consider his physical and mental status so that interventions don't worsen existing problems or create new ones. For example, if your patient needs the support of two nurses during frequent ambulation, include that information in your intervention. If you're teaching a patient to perform a new exercise, make sure he can do the exercise without hurting or straining himself.

Follow the policies of your health care facility

Your interventions must conform with facility policies. If your facility has a rule that only nurses may administer medications, don't write an intervention calling for the patient to administer hemorrhoidal suppositories as needed.

Take other health care activities into account

You're responsible for coordinating nursing care around other scheduled activities, which sometimes may interfere with your nursing interventions. For example, you may want your patient to get plenty of rest on a day he has several diagnostic tests scheduled. Therefore, you may need to reschedule such activities as exercises, support groups, or patient teaching.

Include available resources

To help carry out interventions effectively, make full use of your facility's resources and outside sources, such as support groups. For example, if a patient with a peptic ulcer needs to learn more about necessary dietary and life-style changes, provide him with literature and teaching videotapes or audiotapes, answer questions, and refer him to appropriate outside resources, such as the National Ulcer Foundation.

Writing the intervention statement

When writing interventions, state the necessary action clearly. Many interventions must be continued—and possibly evaluated and modified—by other nurses when you're not present. Also, if your patient and his family are participating in his care, they'll need to understand the intervention. To ensure continuity of care and clear communication, write your interventions in precise detail. Include how and when to perform the intervention as well as any special instructions.

For example, the intervention "Change body position" is vague because it can be interpreted in several ways and doesn't tell another nurse which actions to take. In contrast, "Turn and position patient every 2 hours and provide meticulous skin care" provides specific instructions. Or you could write: "Place patient in lateral or prone position and change position at least every 2 hours." (Note that both statements are ways to interpret "Change body position" but that each has a different rationale. The first is to prevent skin breakdown; the second, to reduce the aspiration risk by allowing secretions and blood to drain. Writing a more specific intervention reduces the potential for such confusion.)

DOCUMENTING THE PLAN OF CARE

Historically, the plan of care was used only by the nursing staff; it was discarded when the patient was discharged and wasn't considered part of the permanent medical record. However, in 1991, the Joint Commission on Accreditation of Healthcare Organizations (JCAHO) mandated that the plan of care must be permanently integrated into the patient's medical record by written or electronic means.

JCAHO policy changes have also led to greater flexibility when planning care. The JCAHO no longer specifies the format for documenting patient care. As a result, new documentation methods have emerged that can make planning faster and easier. This section describes both the traditional and standardized plan of care. Newer, alternative formats for documenting care, including protocols and critical paths, are also discussed.

Using a traditional plan

The traditional plan of care is written from scratch for each patient. Formats vary, but most include three main columns: one for nursing diagnoses, another for expected outcomes, and a third for interventions. A place may also be provided for you to enter the date you initiated the plan, the target dates for expected outcomes, and dates for review, revision, and resolution.

This type of plan is highly specific and can be tailored easily to the individual patient and health care facility. However, because it's typically handwritten, it may be hard to read and to preserve on microfilm. Also, for the patient with an extended hospital stay, a traditional plan may become too lengthy or cumbersome to work with. You may find a traditional plan time-consuming to maintain and may be tempted to place it at the bottom of a pile of papers if you're burdened with documentation. (See *Documenting a traditional plan of care*, page 116.)

Using a standardized plan

The standardized plan of care was developed in response to problems associated with the traditional plan of care. This format provides preprinted information that is not included with a traditional plan — for example, a standardized plan may provide specific nursing diagnoses, outcome statements, and recommended interventions — along with blank spaces. To individualize the plan for your patient, you would fill in the etiologic statement, document signs and symptoms, write in

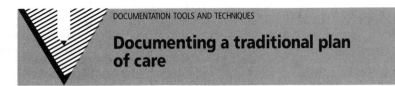

DOCUMENTATION TOOLS AND TECHNIQUES

Documenting a traditional plan of care

In a traditional plan of care, such as the sample shown below, you must write out all information.

Patient's name: *Preston Fielding III*				
Date	Nursing diagnosis	Expected outcomes	Interventions	Review (initials and date)
6/16/93	Ineffective family coping related to caring for an aging, dependent family member.	Family members express feelings about responsibilities of caring for an older relative by end of year	• Educate patient and family members about aging process. Discuss how changes in patient have affected the family. • Arrange and conduct a conference for family members; include patient when possible. • Encourage family members to express their feelings about caring for an older family member.	
		Patient and family members locate appropriate community services by 8/31/93	Assist patient and family members in deciding whether to seek help and in identifying appropriate community services, such as adult day care, respite care, and geriatric outreach services.	
				M.F. 6/16/93

target dates for expected outcomes, and specify intervals and special instructions for interventions. The plan may also provide blank spaces to write evaluation data and resolution dates for expected outcomes. (See *Documenting a standardized plan of care*, pages 118 and 119.)

Most standardized plans are created by hospital-wide committees. They reflect each facility's documentation standards and, through use and review, may reveal areas of nursing care that need improvement.

Standardized plans are now the most common format used. They require far less writing than traditional plans. They're also more legible and easier to duplicate and preserve on microfilm. Besides saving you time, they promote compliance with facility policy and make it easier for novice and ancillary staff to follow the plan of care. They guide you in creating the plan while giving you the flexibility to adapt it to your patient.

However, standardized plans do have some drawbacks. If you yield to the temptation simply to check off items on a list or fill in blanks, you may fail to individualize care or document findings to the extent necessary. A unit-based quality assurance program, which encourages staff members to become involved in audits of plans of care, can help prevent these problems.

Using a protocol
A newer documentation tool, a protocol gives specific sequential instructions for treating patients with a particular problem. Originally, protocols were developed to guide nurses in using equipment or performing specific procedures. Now, they're also used to manage patients according to nursing diagnosis. Protocols may supplement a traditional or standardized plan of care; they may also be used alone to demonstrate planned care.

Protocols offer many advantages. They make it easier to meet hospital administration requirements for providing detailed documentation. Because they spell out the steps to follow for all patients with a particular nursing diagnosis, they help ensure that each patient receives consistent care from all caregivers. For this reason, they can prove invaluable in facilities that rely heavily on inexperienced or technical staff, serving as an on-the-job training tool. (One possible disadvantage of protocols is that they may discourage advanced practitioners from using autonomy and flexibility when providing care.)

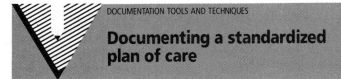

DOCUMENTATION TOOLS AND TECHNIQUES

Documenting a standardized plan of care

You'll find below a sample standardized plan of care. To customize this plan for your patient, you'd check off the relevant terms and phrases and add information where appropriate.

Patient's name
Derrick
Evans

Date
2/10/94

Nursing diagnosis
High risk for peripheral neurovascular dysfunction related to:
- ☐ Trauma
- ☐ Traction (skeletal or musculoskeletal)
- ☑ Cast, splint, or brace
- ☐ Dislocation, subluxation, or fracture
- ☐ Impaired peripheral circulation
- ☑ Other *surgery, rt. wrist*

Assessment findings
Add laboratory findings, observations, or other relevant clinical data in space provided.
- ☑ Pulses (radial, ulnar, brachial, femoral, popliteal, posterior tibial, dorsalis pedis) *evaluate q4 hours*
- ☑ Capillary refill time *evaluate q4 hours*
- ☑ Skin color and temperature *evaluate q4 hours*
- ☑ Pain (specify constant or intermittent; if intermittent, specify stationary or with movement) *evaluate q4 hours*
- ☑ Range of motion *limited*
- ☑ Tactile sensation in extremity *evaluate q4 hours*
- ☐ Alignment of extremity
- ☐ Other

Target dates
2/12/94

5/01/94

2/20/94

2/20/94

Expected outcomes
1. Patient demonstrates improved circulation in extremities, as evidenced by normal, easily located pulses; capillary refill time less than or equal to 2 seconds; improved appearance of extremity; absence of paresthesia; correct extremity alignment; and absence of pain.
2. Patient doesn't experience diminished sensory or motor function in extremity.
3. Patient shows improved range of motion (specify). *in rt. hand*
4. Additional expected outcomes: *Patient regains sensation in digits*

Documenting a standardized plan of care – *continued*

Interventions
• Assess pulse, capillary refill time, sensation, and range of motion of patient's *rt. hand* (specify extremity) every *24 hours*.

• Assess for presence or absence of pain or paresthesia.
• Maintain correct alignment of affected extremity.
• Assess fit of immobilizer, casts, braces, or traction (circle one).
• Inject neurotoxic drugs away from extremity and major nerves.
• Avoid flexing extremity.
• Administer and monitor vasodilators (specify), as ordered. *N/A*

• Instruct patient and caregiver in proper positions for lying in bed and sitting and for relieving pressure.
• Instruct patient and caregiver in how to recognize signs and symptoms of peripheral neurovascular dysfunction, including numbness, pain, and tingling.
• Additional interventions: *Check for infection at surgical site. Discuss cause of injury and preventative measures with patient.*

A protocol also may spell out the role of other health care professionals, such as nursing assistants and staff from other departments. This helps all team members coordinate their efforts.

Using a protocol can save you a lot of documentation time. For example, in the interventions section of a plan of care, you can note that you'll follow a certain protocol by writing "Follow telemetry protocol." (However, a potential drawback is that staff members following the plan of care may fail to go to the appropriate source to read the protocol.)

When choosing a protocol for your patient, be sure to select the one that best fits his needs. Modify interventions as necessary, delete any interventions that don't apply, and update the protocol as the patient's condition changes. (See *Following a patient care protocol,* pages 120 to 122.)

(Text continues on page 122.)

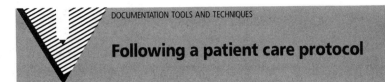

Following a patient care protocol

The sample below shows a patient care protocol. This documentation tool gives specific instructions for providing thorough, consistent care.

Nursing diagnosis: Decreased cardiac output

Responsibilities of the health care team
- Assessment: RN, LPN
- Planning: RN
- Intervention: RN, LPN, nursing assistant
- Patient teaching: RN, dietitian
- Complications: RN
- Evaluation: RN
- Documentation: RN, LPN, dietitian

Caregiver skills
The caregiver must:
- demonstrate the ability to identify arrhythmias correctly and treat them appropriately
- be able to assess the patient's cardiovascular status
- possess appropriate qualifications and certifications, as outlined by hospital policy.

Expected outcomes
The patient will:
- remain free from arrhythmias and other signs of decreased cardiac output
- identify factors that increase risk of cardiac disease, such as lack of exercise, high-fat diet, stress, obesity, and excessive alcohol intake
- identify signs and symptoms of decreased cardiac output and know when and how to obtain medical help if necessary
- demonstrate knowledge of how to restrict sodium intake to 2 g daily through appropriate selection from hospital menu.

Supportive assessment findings
Presence of risk factors
- Family history of heart disease
- Diet high in cholesterol and fat
- Sedentary life-style, infrequent exercise
- Cigarette smoking
- Obesity
- High alcohol intake
Signs and symptoms of myocardial irritability
- Symptomatic arrhythmias resulting in chest pain, nausea, syncope, or diaphoresis
- Electrocardiogram (ECG) demonstrating arrhythmia

Following a patient care protocol – *continued*

Responsibility	Nursing actions

Assessment	• Apply telemetry monitoring system.
	  – Explain the monitoring system and its purpose to patient.
	  – Clean selected sites on chest wall with alcohol; then dry them completely.
	  – Apply telemetry pads to the lead areas most reflective of patient's disease.
	  – Teach patient not to get system wet.
	• Assess patient's cardiopulmonary status every 4 hours or more often if necessary.
	• Assess activity tolerance every 8 hours or more often if necessary.
	• Assess chest pain by identifying the following characteristics:
	  – location and presence or absence of radiation
	  – severity (have patient rate severity on a scale of 1 to 10, with 1 being little pain and 10 being the worst pain he's ever experienced)
	  – duration, onset, method of relief
	  – character (crushing, squeezing, or heaviness).

Planning	• Collaborate with doctor, patient, and family to manage patient's cardiac disease and decrease risk factors. • Meet with dietitian to arrange patient teaching that will reinforce nursing and medical directions.

Interventions	• Establish an I.V. line.
	  – Explain purpose of I.V. line to patient.
	  – Insert heparin lock, preferably avoiding dorsal surface of hand, which is unsuitable for some medications (such as diazepam and phenytoin).
	• Maintain I.V. line patency with heparin flushes (10 units) every shift and as necessary.
	• Monitor ECG for arrhythmias.
	• Assess patient for chest pain.
	• Auscultate heart and breath sounds to detect changes in cardiopulmonary status.
	• Monitor laboratory values, especially electrolyte and cardiac enzyme levels.
	• Measure patient's weight and intake and output.
	• Observe patient activity. Correlate presence or absence of chest pain, arrhythmias, or shortness of breath with activity.
	• Administer prescribed medications, as ordered.
	• Assess effectiveness of medications.

(continued)

Following a patient care protocol – *continued*

Responsibility	Nursing actions
Patient and family teaching	• Explain pathophysiology in simple terms to patient and family. • Explain the action and desired effects of prescribed medications to patient and family. • Teach family members how to perform cardiopulmonary resuscitation correctly. • Explain extent and purpose of activity restrictions. • Teach patient and family how and when to get medical help in case of emergency, unrelieved chest pain, or shortness of breath.
Recognition of complications	• Observe for complications, including: — symptomatic arrhythmias — hypotension — hypokalemia — cardiac arrest — congestive heart failure.
Evaluation	• Evaluate cardiac status by continuous cardiac monitoring. • Assess effectiveness of antiarrhythmic medication. • Evaluate patient's readiness to learn and his knowledge level.
Documentation	• Document the following: — presence or absence of arrhythmias q 4 hours — episodes of chest pain (including pain characteristics) — presence of other signs and symptoms of decreased cardiac output — location and patency of I.V. lines q 4 hours — vital signs q 4 hours and as needed — ECG strips q 4 hours and as needed — intake and output q 8 hours — medication administration — daily weight, vital signs, and intake and output on graphic sheets — activity tolerance — complications and corrective actions taken.

Using a critical path

A critical path is used in hospitals that use a case management system for delivering care. In this system, a registered nurse is responsible for managing a closely monitored and controlled system of multidisciplinary care and must assume responsibility for outcomes, length of stay, and use of equipment throughout the patient's illness. The case management approach to delivering health care developed in response to the diagnosis-related group (DRG) system introduced by the federal government in 1983. Under the DRG system, the government stipulates in advance how much it will reimburse a hospital under Medicare. Reimbursement hinges primarily on the patient's medical diagnosis (other factors such as age and complications are considered). Each diagnosis receives a DRG code number. Note that payment is determined without regard to the patient's length of stay or the number or types of services he receives. Thus, the facility loses money if it costs more to treat the patient than Medicare will pay under the DRG system.

As a tool for managed care, the critical path may provide an alternative method for documenting nursing activities. Typically, a critical path includes the patient's medical diagnosis, the length of stay allowed under the DRG system, expected outcomes, and key events that must occur for the patient to be discharged by the target date. Such events may include consultations, diagnostic tests, physical activities the patient must perform, treatments, diet, medications, discharge planning, and patient teaching. Besides long- and short-term goals, a critical path outlines nurse-doctor collaboration. (See *Following a critical path,* pages 124 and 125.)

With critical paths, you're likely to use facility resources more efficiently and achieve patient resolution target dates matching those mandated by the DRG. If your patient needs a longer stay, the justification becomes part of his hospital record.

A drawback of critical paths is that they take a long time to develop as nursing tools. The practitioner must be able to recognize when deviations from the path are necessary; therefore, use of critical paths is restricted to registered nurses. Implementation of a documentation system that relies on critical paths requires a strong commitment on the part of hospital administrators. Use of critical paths may be discontinued by administrators because of cost and failure to recognize the benefits of increasing the role of the professional nursing staff. Resistance may also be encountered from some medical staff members, who view implementation of critical paths as a step toward increased autonomous practice for nurses.

(Text continues on page 126.)

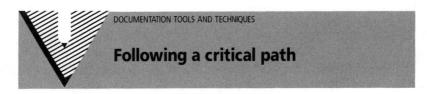

DOCUMENTATION TOOLS AND TECHNIQUES

Following a critical path

The sample below shows you selected portions of a typical critical path, starting with the preoperative day and continuing through the first two postoperative days.

CRITICAL PATH

Diagnosis: Partial or total parotidectomy
DRG length of stay: 2.3 days
Actual length of stay: _2.3 days_

Expected outcomes
By discharge, the patient will:
• state possible complications, troubleshooting measures, and appropriate resources
• perform suture line care
• discuss measures for managing his pain
• explain how to maintain his nutritional status.

Nurse	Other health care providers	Patient and family
Preoperative day		
• Performs assessment • Explains case management model and recovery pathway to patient • Completes contract with patient and family • Performs preoperative teaching • Notifies social worker, if appropriate, and explains assessment and possible discharge needs to her	*Primary doctor* • Performs physical examination • Orders special studies, including blood work, electrocardiogram, and chest X-rays • Orders anesthesia clearance assessment *Social worker* • Consults with nurse (if appropriate)	*Patient and family* • Sign contract • Visit postoperative care unit

Following a critical path – *continued*

Nurse	Other health care providers	Patient and family
Postoperative day 1		
• Provides morning care while patient is on bed rest • Sets up heparin lock on I.V. line • Teaches suture line care • Teaches eye care (if applicable) • Encourages activity • Monitors diet	*Primary doctor* • Orders laboratory tests • Orders advance in diet as tolerated • Orders heparin lock on I.V. line • Consults with ophthalmologist, radiation therapist, and dentist (if applicable) *Ophthalmologist* • Consults with doctor (if applicable) *Radiation therapist* • Consults with doctor (if applicable) *Dentist* • Consults with doctor (if applicable)	*Patient* • Performs oral hygiene and incentive spirometry • Demonstrates suture line care and eye care (if applicable) • Ambulates q 4 hr p.r.n.
Postoperative day 2		
• Continues to teach suture line care and eye care • Continues to encourage activity and monitor diet	*Dietitian* • Performs nutrition assessment *Speech pathologist* • Performs speech assessment (if patient has difficulty swallowing)	*Patient* • Performs morning self-care • Continues to perform oral hygiene and incentive spirometry • Demonstrates suture line care • Ambulates q 4 hr p.r.n.

• When planning your patient's care, you must establish care priorities, develop expected outcomes, formulate nursing interventions, and document the plan in the appropriate format.

• The plan of care is a dynamic record that must be reviewed daily and revised according to the patient's progress and changes in the treatment regimen.

• The plan of care provides a central source of information for members of the health care team.

• Maslow's hierarchy of needs is a system of classifying human needs that may prove helpful when seeking to establish care priorities for patients with multiple nursing diagnoses.

• Involving your patient and family members in planning is crucial to ensuring successful nursing care.

• Expected outcomes are measurable, patient-focused goals that are derived from the patient's nursing diagnoses. They should be written in precise, quantitative terms and should focus on patient behaviors, not nursing actions.

• When developing interventions for your patient, focus on the etiologic portion of the diagnostic statement, keep your patient's safety in mind, tailor the intervention to your patient's circumstances, follow the policies of your health care facility, take other health care activities into account, and include available resources.

• JCAHO policy changes have led to greater flexibility when planning care. The JCAHO no longer specifies the format for documenting patient care. As a result, new documentation methods have emerged that can speed and simplify planning.

• Standardized plans of care provide some preprinted information along with blank spaces. Now the most common format used, standardized plans require far less writing than traditional plans. They're also more legible and easier to duplicate and preserve on microfilm.

• A newer documentation tool, protocols give sequential instructions for treating patients with a specific nursing diagnosis. Protocols make it easier to meet hospital administration requirements for providing detailed documentation and can help ensure that the patient receives consistent care from all caregivers.

SELF-TEST

1. The plan of care includes:
    a. patient assessment data, the medical treatment plan, and diagnostic test results.
    b. doctor's orders, operative proceedings, and medication administration.
    c. the collected documentation of all team members providing care for your patient.
    d. the patient's nursing diagnoses, expected outcomes, nursing interventions, teaching plan, and evaluation data.

2. Who should have access to the plan of care?
    a. nursing staff only
    b. the nurse, patient, and family
    c. the doctor and nurse
    d. all caregivers, plus the patient and family

3. When setting care priorities, you should assign the highest priority to life-threatening problems and the lowest priority to:
    a. safety-related needs.
    b. needs that are not related to the patient's specific illness or prognosis.
    c. the patient's emotional (love and belonging) needs.
    d. needs of family members and friends who are involved in the patient's care.

4. Which statement best describes Maslow's hierarchy of human needs?
    a. It focuses on the need of all human beings to belong to a family or group.
    b. It implies that human beings rarely have the means to satisfy all of their physiologic needs and that they inevitably encounter conflict when seeking to address higher-level needs.
    c. It portrays human needs as linear and emphasizes that basic and abstract needs must be met simultaneously.

d. It describes five levels of human needs and stresses that basic physiologic needs must be met before higher-level needs can be addressed.

5. According to Orem's self-care theory, which of the following is the nurse's major goal?

  a. to help the patient achieve self-actualization
  b. to help the patient reach the highest possible level of self-care
  c. to help the patient fulfill the universal need for air, food, and water
  d. to help the patient identify his self-care deficits

6. What's the main purpose of the expected outcome statement?

  a. to describe the behavior the patient is expected to achieve as a result of nursing interventions
  b. to describe the nursing procedures to be administered to the patient
  c. to provide a standard for evaluating the quality of health care delivered to the patient during his hospital stay
  d. to make sure that the patient's treatment does not extend beyond the time allowed under the diagnosis-related group system

7. What are the components of an outcome statement?

  a. nursing action, patient behavior, target date, and conditions under which the behavior occurs
  b. patient behavior, measurement criteria, conditions under which the behavior occurs, and target date
  c. target date, nursing action, measurement criteria, and desired patient behavior
  d. nursing diagnosis, interventions, and expected patient behavior

8. Which guideline is most appropriate when developing nursing interventions?

  a. Choose actions that a nurse can perform without leaving the unit or consulting with medical staff.
  b. Make your intervention statements specific to ensure continuity of care.
  c. Write interventions in general terms to allow maximum flexibility and creativity in delivering nursing care.

d. Make sure that nursing care activities receive priority over other aspects of the treatment regimen.

9. Compared to a standardized plan of care, a traditional plan is:

a. easier to preserve on microfilm
b. easier to adapt to recent policy changes by the Joint Commission on Accreditation of Healthcare Organizations (JCAHO)
c. easier to tailor to the individual patient
d. easier to work with, especially when pressed for time

10. Which of the following guidelines is most useful when seeking to develop an effective plan of care?

a. Follow JCAHO requirements carefully; they are intended to guide you step-by-step through the planning process.
b. Avoid imposing too rigid a structure on nursing activities. Caring works best when it's spontaneous.
c. Use newer, up-to-date documentation formats, such as the protocol, instead of the traditional plan of care, which is outdated and cumbersome to document.
d. Establish realistic goals for the patient, individualize your approach to each patient's care, and avoid vague terminology.

(For answers with rationales, turn to page 262.)

FURTHER READINGS

Accreditation Manual for Hospitals. Chicago: Joint Commission on Accreditation of Healthcare Organizations, 1992.

Applebaum, R., and Austin, C. *Long-term Care Case Management: Design and Evaluation.* New York: Springer Publishing Co., 1990.

Benner, P. *From Novice to Expert: Excellence and Power in Clinical Nursing Practice.* Menlo Park, Calif.: Addison-Wesley Publishing Co., 1984.

Cassidy, D., and Friesen, M. "QA: Applying JCAHO's Generic Model," *Nursing Management* 21(6):22-27, June 1990.

Chinn, P., and Kramer, M. *Theory and Nursing: A Systematic Approach,* 3rd ed. St. Louis: Mosby-Year Book, Inc., 1991.

Doenges, M., and Moorehouse, M. *Application of Nursing Process and Nursing Diagnosis: An Interactive Text.* Philadelphia: F.A. Davis Co., 1992.

Eliopoulos, C. *Nursing Care Planning Guides for Long-term Care,* 3rd ed. Baltimore: Williams & Wilkins Co., 1990.

Iyer, P., et al. *Nursing Process and Nursing Diagnosis.* Philadelphia: W.B. Saunders Co., 1991.

Jaffe, M. *Medical-Surgical Nursing Care Plans: Nursing Diagnosis and Interventions,* 2nd ed. East Norwalk, Conn.: Appleton & Lange, 1992.

Leuner, J., et al. *Mastering the Nursing Process: A Case Method Approach.* Philadelphia: F.A. Davis Co., 1990.

Marrelli, T. *Nursing Documentation Handbook.* St. Louis: Mosby-Year Book Inc., 1992.

Mayer, G., et al. *Patient Care Delivery Models.* Gaithersburg, Md.: Aspen Pubs., Inc., 1990.

McElroy, D., and Herbelin, K. "Writing a Better Patient Care Plan," *Nursing88* 18(2):50-51, February 1988.

McRae, M. "Care Plan for the Patient Undergoing Intracardiac Myxoma Excision," *Critical Care Nurse* 10(9):58-60, October 1990.

Orem, D. *Nursing: Concepts of Practice,* 4th ed. New York: McGraw-Hill Book Co., 1991.

Sanford, J., and Disch, J. *AACN Standards for Nursing Care of the Critically Ill,* 2nd ed. East Norwalk, Conn.: Appleton & Lange, 1989.

Short, N., and Bair, L. "Standards of Care: Practicing What We Preach," *Nursing Management* 21(6):32-39, June 1990.

Turner, S. "Nursing Process, Nursing Diagnoses, and Care Plans in a Clinical Setting," *Journal of Nursing Staff Development* 7(5):239-43, September-October, 1991.

Zander, K. "Nursing Case Management: Strategic Management of Cost and Quality Outcomes," *Journal of Nursing Administration* 18(5):23-30, May 1988.

Zander, K., and Etheredge, M., eds. *Collaborative Care: Nursing Case Management.* Chicago: American Hospital Association, 1989.

IMPLEMENTATION

During the fourth phase of the nursing process, you put your plan of care into action. Simply put, you'll *intervene*. Your interventions will help meet your patient's health care needs. They reflect your agreement with the patient on how to help him reach defined goals, or expected outcomes.

This chapter begins by classifying interventions and describing the most common ones. It goes on to address the practical problems you encounter during implementation. You'll find practical advice on how to manage your time wisely and communicate assertively and effectively with colleagues. The chapter ends with techniques for documenting nursing interventions.

CLASSIFYING NURSING INTERVENTIONS

You can classify nursing interventions in various ways. Considering these classifications can help you attain a clearer understanding of nursing practice.

Physiologic, psychological, and socioeconomic interventions

Physiologic interventions help to meet the patient's basic needs, including oxygen, food, water, elimination, sleep, and comfort. You may need to use special equipment, such as a nasal cannula or a urinary catheter, to satisfy physiologic needs.

Psychological interventions seek to enhance the patient's emotional well-being. These include allowing the patient to express his feelings, dimming room light, and arranging for the patient to have at his bedside personal items that provide comfort.

Socioeconomic interventions are geared toward enhancing the patient's overall quality of life. Examples include referring a homeless patient to an emergency shelter or appropriate social service agencies, or assessing a patient's financial and insurance status to determine if he meets eligibility requirements for receiving aid from government or community resources.

Sometimes you'll find that your actions will meet several of the patient's needs simultaneously. For example, a physiologic intervention, such as therapeutic touch, can relax the patient, thus providing a psychological benefit.

Independent, dependent, and interdependent interventions

Independent interventions are actions you initiate without the direction of a doctor or other member of the health care team. Although you usually determine and implement these interventions independently, you may also coordinate them with other care activities. Examples include helping the patient with activities of daily living, counseling, and patient teaching.

Dependent interventions are based on written or oral instructions provided by a doctor or other member of the health care team. Examples include preparing and administering medication, inserting an indwelling urinary catheter, and obtaining a specimen for laboratory tests.

Interdependent, or *collaborative*, interventions are planned jointly by members of the health care team. Carrying out interdependent interventions requires your knowledge, judgment, and discretion. Examples include carrying out standing orders or following a protocol.

Alternative classification

At the 1992 conference of the North American Nursing Diagnosis Association (NANDA), Bulechek and McCloskey suggested another scheme for classifying nursing interventions:
• nurse-initiated actions in response to a nursing diagnosis
• doctor-initiated actions in response to a medical diagnosis
• assistance with the patient's daily functioning or with activities that aren't directly related to a nursing or medical diagnosis.

UNDERSTANDING TYPES OF INTERVENTIONS

You may develop ideas for interventions in several ways. For instance, you could consider activities that you or your patient have found helpful in the past. You could also consult with colleagues; refer to textbooks, journal articles, policy and procedure manuals, and unit-specific protocols; or, simply, brainstorm. As long as you remain within the bounds of nursing practice standards, the only limitations are your own creativity, insight, and professional and personal resources. Below are examples of the types of interventions you may perform when providing patient care.

Assessing and monitoring
These interventions are fundamental but significant nursing activities. Periodic or continuous evaluation of your patient's condition and response to an intervention is just as important as the initial assessment. Examples of these interventions include recording vital signs, such as pulse rate, on a regular basis (such as every 4 hours) and reporting irregularities; observing the patient for adverse reactions to drugs; or obtaining specimens for monitoring laboratory test values.

Providing therapeutic care
These interventions are geared toward curing the patient's illness or restoring optimal function. You may provide, supervise, or coordinate therapeutic interventions. For example, if you administer medications, you're performing a therapeutic intervention for restoring health. On the other hand, you may coordinate physical, respiratory, or occupational therapy aimed at the same goal but provided by other health care workers. Other therapeutic interventions include suctioning to stimulate a cough and clear airways, administering oxygen, providing range-of-motion exercises, and performing wound care.

Promoting comfort and function
You or your patient may initiate these goal-directed, independent interventions. Additionally, you may involve other members of the health care team as well as members of the patient's family. For example, you could ease stress placed on the patient by asking one family member to call the patient at specified times and relay messages from him to other family members.

Supporting respiration and elimination
Supporting these functions is essential for your patient's well-being. For example, you may enhance the patient's chest expansion by assisting him to a comfortable position, such as leaning on an overbed table with a pillow. You may also help the patient with constipation establish a defecation routine by placing him on a bedpan or commode at a specific time daily, as close to his usual defecation time (if known) as possible.

Providing skin care

Proper skin care helps maintain skin integrity and prevent pressure ulcers. Examples of nursing measures include turning the patient to avoid skin breakdown and providing a prescribed regimen to treat the underlying skin condition.

Managing the environment

Work to ensure privacy and provide a comfortable, therapeutic environment for the patient. Begin by minimizing noise to ensure a good night's sleep. Arrange for the patient to have at the bedside objects that provide spiritual comfort (Bible, prayer shawl, pictures, statues, rosary beads). Provide privacy during the patient's visits with a clergyman. Identify and reduce unnecessary stimuli in the environment.

Providing food and fluids

This type of intervention may include encouraging a special diet, such as a high-potassium, low-sodium, or low-cholesterol diet. Other examples include reviewing your patient's dietary habits, administering total parenteral nutrition, initiating oral intake, and providing nutritional counseling.

Giving emotional support

You may plan and implement interventions to enhance a patient's emotional well-being, taking into account physiologic, emotional, social, sexual, or financial concerns. For example, you may encourage the patient to express feelings about his condition and its effect on family members; schedule a specific time to talk with the patient; and take steps to establish a trusting, supportive relationship.

Teaching and counseling

Teaching helps your patient maintain his health and avoid future problems. For example, if your patient experiences post-traumatic stress disorder as a result of an assault, you may counsel him on ways to seek support from others when frightened. You might also provide the patient and his family members with information about managing physical injuries, tailoring your instructions to the patient's capacity to learn.

Providing referrals

Self-help and other support groups have gained popularity in the past decade because they provide people with needed support outside their existing social networks. Support groups may promote changes in behavior (Co-dependents Anonymous, for example), provide support for families (Al-Anon), or focus on a specific illness (Alzheimer's Association) or life-style (Parents without Partners). Other sources of support may include senior citizen centers and community services, such as Meals On Wheels and home health care agencies. To help patients and any family members who might benefit from one of these groups, find out which services are available from your health care facility and from outside sources, then develop a core of support services. (For more information, see *Self-help option*, page 136.)

INTERVENING
Intervention, or implementation, overlaps with all other phases of the nursing process. For instance, when you provide care, you'll also evaluate your patient's responses to the interventions, reassess the interventions, and review and modify sections of the plan of care as needed.

Understand the rationale for each intervention
Always consider the rationale—the fundamental reason behind each intervention. Understanding rationales can improve critical thinking and help avoid mistakes. It can also make repetitive or sometimes unappealing interventions more interesting.

Be aware of possible adverse effects
Not only should you know the expected effect of each intervention, you should also be able to anticipate and recognize potentially harmful adverse effects.

Involve family members
When possible, let family members participate in the patient's care. This will help support the patient and help preserve the family unit's integrity. If, however, the family's dysfunctional coping patterns prevent them from participating, you must learn to accept their limitations. Dysfunctional family coping patterns evolve over many years and are unlikely to change just because one member of the family has a serious illness. Accepting the family's behavior will help you avoid burnout and better meet the patient's needs.

Self-help option

During the past decade, support groups have proliferated. Besides the long-standing support groups for alcoholics and drug abusers, support groups now exist for incest survivors, stutterers, burn victims, suicide survivors, patients with Parkinson's disease, and many others.

This rapid growth in support groups can be attributed to several factors: a more open society and media exposure of once-taboo subjects, such as incest and child abuse; increased self-awareness and a growing sense of empowerment among patients; frustration with conventional methods of obtaining help; and a general trend toward self-improvement. When formulating interventions for your patient, consider whether a support group would be beneficial. Keep the following points in mind when incorporating support groups in your plan of care:

• Consider the patient's needs, strengths, and weaknesses, and carefully match them with the appropriate support group. Determine if your patient needs the added support of a group, if he will benefit from the support group atmosphere, and if he will feel comfortable sharing his thoughts and feelings with others.

• Recommend support groups as a supplement to treatment — not as a substitute for it.

• If appropriate, investigate how family, friends, co-workers, and religious groups can provide a support structure as well.

• If your patient refuses to attend a support group, assess whether he can help himself without the group or if he's just denying his problem and feelings.

• Consider the patient's nursing diagnoses when determining the need for a support group. Patients with such diagnoses as *social isolation, spiritual distress, rape-trauma syndrome, posttrauma response, altered role performance, ineffective individual coping, ineffective family coping, caregiver role strain,* and *impaired social interaction* commonly make excellent candidates for support groups.

• Find out which support services are available in your institution and the patient's community. Consult members of the health care team, community telephone directories, and social service agencies, and talk to support group leaders or attend their meetings.

• If your patient joins a support group, plan a follow-up meeting to discuss whether his effort was successful. Ask the patient if he's satisfied with the group. Periodically assess whether the group is meeting his needs: Is the patient's stress reduced? Is he making any progress toward achieving his goals? Ask the patient if he wants to remain in the group.

Perform periodic reassessments

Periodically reassess your nursing interventions to ascertain whether they're still appropriate for attaining expected outcomes and to determine if any interventions need to be modified or discontinued.

Identify needed skills and knowledge

Evaluate your ability to perform nursing interventions. If necessary, seek additional information or obtain help from nursing colleagues or other experts in your facility.

Increase professional effectiveness

During implementation, you usually have the most direct and prolonged contact with the patient. You must also coordinate and direct the activities of other members of the health care team. To ensure successful care of your patient, evaluate the quality of your nursing practice and focus on maximizing your effectiveness—for example, by following the suggestions described below.

Time management

Learning to use time wisely can increase your effectiveness and efficiency. For guidelines to good time management, remember the acronym PACE:
• **P**lan your day.
• **A**ssess your patients.
• **C**are for your patients and yourself.
• **E**nd your shift on time.

Plan your day

Before you report, set up a time sheet listing each hour of your shift; leave enough space for notes after each heading. This sheet will help you organize the work that needs to be completed at scheduled times. You'll find it especially useful when you have to juggle care for many patients.

When you record histories, assessments, medication orders, and treatments for patients on your regular report sheet, jot down notes on the time sheet. Remember that you're using the time sheet as a quick reference tool to remind you of things that you need to do (or make sure that others do). Don't put every bit of information on the time sheet or it will be too cluttered to be useful.

As you step onto the unit, no matter how hectic it is, keep calm as you continue to formulate a plan for your day. Check on any outstanding orders or preoperative schedules, and stay organized by adding them to your time sheet. Although emergencies or requests for pain medications may disrupt your schedule, always return to your plan.

Assess your patients

Making a patient assessment round before you provide care is is a good practice to adopt and it will save time. Because you won't have time to assess each patient fully, focus on the reason for the patient's hospitalization. If the patient had back surgery, examine his incision line and ask how his back feels. Remember, you can do a more thorough assessment later.

Except for emergencies, don't stop for extensive care. Of course, if a patient needs a bedpan, you'll want to get it right away. But if someone asks for help getting up and dressed, explain that you'll be back to help him as soon as you finish doing a quick check on all of your patients.

Care for your patients and yourself

Because this step will involve the majority of your day, make sure you establish priorities, delegate tasks, and care for yourself to help control your time.

Although you may have a plan and certain tasks that you need to finish, be flexible. You may expect to spend only 10 minutes with a patient, but if he's in physical or emotional distress, you may need to stay longer. As your plan changes, you need to establish priorities—decide which situations require attention before others. This skill improves with experience. If you're new, ask a more experienced nurse which situation should take precedence over another and why.

Managing time efficiently sometimes requires delegating tasks to others. On some units and for some nurses, delegation proves difficult. If you have trouble delegating, ask yourself why. Do those working with you refuse to accept delegation? Do they manipulate you? Do they manipulate others? If you answer yes to any of these questions, ask for your nurse-manager's help in working through these problems.

Examine your own attitude about asking for help. Do you feel uncomfortable asking for help? Would you rather try doing everything yourself? If so, you need to work on changing your attitude. Remember that failing to delegate when appropriate is counterproductive in the long run. For example, you might have time to take a specimen to the laboratory today, but coworkers may expect you to continue this practice even when you no longer have time. Besides, those minutes might be better spent planning care or talking to a patient.

Don't neglect your own needs. Insist on breaks and time for lunch. Don't try to remain in high gear physically and emotionally all day. When you do take a break, try to get away from the unit—and don't talk about your patients.

Don't take on more than you can handle. When you're busy, don't let others delegate to you. You can say no when time constraints make it necessary.

End your shift on time
Sometimes, despite your best efforts, you may find that leaving work on time is difficult. Charting and reporting are two common holdups.

If charting is a problem and you have a few minutes of free time during your shift, start to chart your patients' assessments and progress. You can always add notes later to reflect any changes in your patients' conditions.

You may need to ask your nurse-manager to evaluate the report system in your facility. For example, each nurse may be required to know everything about each patient—a policy that may no longer be realistic or cost-effective. Alternative report systems, such as taped or walking reports or silent reports (in which you just read the previous shift's documentation), may help you save time.

Remember that there are three shifts to care for patients. As long as you avoid overloading the next shift, you can justly expect their help in completing unfinished tasks.

Relationships with colleagues
Maintaining smooth working relationships with your colleagues is crucial to the success of your nursing care. Below you'll find advice for learning how to act assertively, handle criticism, and cope with professional conflicts.

Acting assertively
To be assertive, you need to identify goals, act to attain them, and take responsibility for your actions. You should be able to distinguish assertive behavior from aggressive behavior, which is meant to put down others through attacks or threats and which may result from the need to release pent-up emotions brought on by avoiding conflict. (See *Practicing assertiveness*, pages 140 and 141.)

Handling criticism ˙
In working with colleagues, you must learn to give and receive criticism and evaluate its validity. Criticism can be either pos-

Practicing assertiveness

To learn to communicate assertively and effectively, you'll need to practice these steps.

Don't be afraid to say no
If you're already swamped and your nurse-manager asks you to take on more work, just say, "I'd like to help, but I have all the patients I can handle right now." Or you might agree to take on a new patient if your nurse-manager assigns another nurse to one of your present patients. Most important, don't feel guilty about saying no. By refusing to be overburdened, you're doing the right thing not only for yourself but also for your patients.

Say what you mean
Don't wait around hoping people will figure out what you want. Instead, state exactly what you're after. For example, if you're interested in working in a different department, say, "I'd like to be transferred to the oncology department" rather than "I understand the oncology department is a great place to work."

Confront others directly
Assertive behavior is characterized by ownership of feelings and needs. Statements such as "I think," "I need," or "I'm angry" reflect ownership and accountability.

Learn to listen
When someone is talking to you, pay attention to what she's saying and how she's saying it. While she's talking, don't try to figure out what she means or what your response is going to be. If you have questions about her meaning, paraphrase what she said to make sure that what you heard is what she meant. For example, say, "Let me make sure I understand. You want me to take care of Mrs. Jones in room 303B before I help Mary pass out meds."

If explanations or instructions are ambiguous, ask for clarification. But be careful not to put the other person on the defensive. Say, "I didn't quite understand which assignment you wanted me to tackle first" rather than "You're not making yourself clear."

Watch your body language
Make sure that your body language doesn't conflict with the message you want to convey or the message you're receiving. For instance, don't speak softly and agreeably while leaning forward aggressively. Likewise, don't smile if you're giving or receiving distressing news. These conflicting behaviors send mixed messages; the listener will feel confused and ambivalent. Also, avoid distracting nervous movements, such as wringing your hands, which demonstrate uncertainty and lack of confidence. Always speak firmly in a pleasant, authoritative voice and maintain good eye contact. But don't overplay your firmness by looking too severe or imposing.

Practicing assertiveness – *continued*

Build self-confidence and a positive self-image
Although modesty is a virtue, it can hold you back when selling yourself or your ideas to your nurse-manager or colleagues. Learn to accept praise when it's appropriate. Don't negate a compliment by saying, "It was nothing." Instead, accept praise gracefully by saying, "Thank you; that's good to hear" or "It was a lot of hard work, but I'm glad you're pleased with the results."

Don't be afraid of rejection
Nobody likes rejection, but it's a part of life. By preparing yourself for the fact that some of your ideas and requests will be turned down, you'll be better able to take the rejection in stride. And you'll be ready to start thinking of new ideas or new ways to move ahead.

---

itive or negative and can range from a compliment to, unfortunately, an insult.

Learning to express criticism constructively fosters teamwork. Constructive criticism is an evaluation of one's performance as a nurse, not a judgment about one's character. When offering criticism to a peer, examine your own motivations, carefully phrase the criticism in an assertive yet nonthreatening manner, and speak privately. Be prepared for acceptance or rejection of your criticism.

Likewise, receiving criticism can enhance self-development. Don't be afraid to seek feedback about your performance from supervisors and colleagues whose opinions you respect. (See *How to give and receive criticism,* page 142.)

Coping with professional conflicts
Working with a variety of people has many benefits: It allows you and your co-workers to learn from each other and makes the job more interesting. But it also leads to conflict. Conflict is inevitable in any organization when people come together with different backgrounds, values, perceptions, and priorities. You probably respond to conflict much the same way each time it occurs. How you handle conflict can affect the way you feel about your career. If you often give in, you may end up frustrated and angry; if you always fight back, you may feel burned out and lonely.

How to give and receive criticism

Consider the following suggestions for giving and receiving criticism.

Giving criticism
• Voice your criticism as soon as possible—don't put it off. Waiting may only add fuel to your fire.
• Make sure that you focus on one thing at a time. Don't overload someone with a list of concerns. And don't repeat a point once you've made it; chances are, the person won't forget what you've said.
• Object only to actions that the other person can change. Asking her to do something she's incapable of doing will only lead to frustration.
• If possible, try to present your criticism as either a suggestion or a question.
• Avoid sarcasm. Sarcasm signals that you're angry at the person—not her actions—and may make her resentful.
• Avoid words such as *always* and *never.* They're usually less than accurate, and defending them can put you in an awkward position.
• Don't apologize for your criticism. Doing so may indicate that you're not sure whether you had the right to say what you did and will only confuse the person you're criticizing.
• Don't forget to use compliments as often as you can. Then when you do criticize, a person will be more likely to accept it.

Receiving criticism
• Buy time. Stop the conversation by saying that you need a couple of minutes to think about what was said or by asking the person to repeat her criticism. This will give you time to think and to compose yourself before you respond.
• Keep your cool. If the other person loses her cool and you're in danger of losing yours, firmly and calmly state that you want to stop the conversation now and resume it when you're both calmer. If necessary, keep saying this until you get through to her.
• Learn new techniques for handling criticism. Suppose the critic is your nurse-manager and she tells you, "You aren't supervising the new student nurse on your unit properly. You've given her too much responsibility too soon. That medication error she made yesterday could have seriously harmed Mr. Roberts." To keep from responding defensively, try one of these techniques:
  — Fogging. Agree with what's true about the criticism, rather than about your actions. You might say, "You're right; the medication error was serious."
  — Negative assertion. Take the steam out of your nurse-manager's critical approach by immediately accepting the negative part of her statement: "I've probably given Mary more responsibility than she's ready to handle."
  — Negative inquiry. When appropriate, ask your nurse-manager to be more specific in her criticism.

Learn to break free from fixed patterns of behavior by tailoring your response to fit the situation. Becoming aware of the five styles used to resolve conflict—competition, accommodation, avoidance, compromise, and collaboration—will help you select the right approach at the right time.

Competition occurs when one person confronts and overpowers another. Aggressive and uncooperative, this approach can leave your adversary feeling angry and belittled.

Accommodation occurs when one person gives in to the other, frequently for the sake of preserving their relationship. This approach is cooperative but unassertive. If you accommodate another person, you may end up feeling anxious and resentful.

With *avoidance*, both parties essentially give up by doing or saying something (such as making a promise but not following through with it) to avoid conflict. Avoidance usually wastes time and creates tension and hard feelings.

The most effective strategies for resolving conflicts are *compromise* and *collaboration*. Compromise occurs when one party agrees to limited behavior modification to achieve resolution; this approach may become problematic if one person compromises too much. Collaboration occurs when both parties agree to modify their behaviors to solve the conflict (see *Handling professional conflicts*, page 144).

Keep the following points in mind as well when deciding how to handle a conflict:

• If you lack any power at all to change a situation, you can't compete, compromise, or collaborate. Instead, you must accommodate or avoid the conflict.

• If you value your relationship with a colleague, try to accommodate, compromise, or collaborate during a conflict. A competitive or avoidance approach may alienate the colleague.

• When you have a lot of time, you can use any of the five techniques. But when you're facing a deadline or an emergency, your best bet is to compete or accommodate. Either way, resolve the conflict quickly, then get on with the task at hand. (A word to the other person later, when you have time, may help ease hurt feelings.)

Collaboration is essential, but may be difficult to achieve, when working with medical staff. Negative social factors may interfere. For example, because nursing is a predominantly female profession, nurses are commonly socialized into being submissive and selfless. They may have been indirectly taught that dealing assertively with doctors and administrators is in-

Handling professional conflicts

How can you resolve a professional conflict effectively? One way is to consider using several strategies, think about their implications, and select the best one, as the following case study demonstrates.

The conflict
Miriam Kantner is a nurse-manager on a 30-bed medical-surgical unit. Soon after Miriam posts next month's schedule, one of her staff nurses says she has to take next Saturday off to attend a relative's wedding. Miriam needs her on Saturday because weekend staffing is low and patient census and acuity are high. Saturday is also Miriam's day off, and she's planning to visit a friend.

Possible strategies
If Miriam were to select competition, she would immediately refuse the nurse's request, explaining that she needs her Saturday because of the expected work load. However, she would have set up a win-lose situation: She would win because she has strengthened her authority, and the staff nurse would lose—both the conflict and some feelings of self-worth.

If Miriam were to select accommodation, she would give the nurse Saturday off and cancel her own plans. This time, she would have set up a lose-win situation: Miriam would lose—she'd probably feel angry when working Saturday—and the nurse would win.

If Miriam were to select avoidance, she would tell the nurse that she'd try to find a replacement, then neglect to follow up. She would avoid conflict by conveniently forgetting the problem. Miriam could hope that the problem would solve itself—that another nurse would ask to work Saturday in exchange for a different day off or that the work load wouldn't be as bad as expected. Probably, she'd become increasingly uncomfortable as the weekend approached. Miriam would have set up a lose-lose situation: She would waste her time and energy dealing with the tension she created by avoiding conflict, and the staff nurse would learn that she can't rely on her manager to come up with an equitable solution.

If Miriam were to select compromise, she would agree to let the nurse leave early enough on Saturday so that she could attend the reception, but she'd have to miss the wedding. Miriam would have created a modified win-lose situation this time: Neither would get exactly what she wants, but neither would be completely disappointed. However, Miriam might still feel uneasy because she would have reduced staffing, even if only for a short time.

Best strategy
If Miriam were to select collaboration, she could propose that the nurse would get Saturday off but would work Sunday and attend a meeting for Miriam on Monday. In exchange, Miriam would work Saturday and visit her friend on Sunday. Here, Miriam would have established a win-win situation: She'd ensure adequate staffing for the entire weekend and still get to travel, and the staff nurse could attend the wedding and the reception.

appropriate. Such factors as financial and educational status, training, and experience level can also be sources of inequity and conflict between doctors and nurses. Additionally, nurses are usually trained to reconcile and negotiate, whereas doctors historically have been trained to be self-reliant, authoritarian, and competitive. (See *Strengthening cooperation between nurses and doctors*, pages 146 and 147.)

DOCUMENTING INTERVENTIONS

You're responsible for documenting each intervention in the patient's clinical record, the time it occurred, your observations, the patient's response, and any other pertinent information. Make sure that each entry relates to a nursing diagnosis. This information becomes a data base for monitoring quality, evaluating the patient's progress, providing continuity of care, and planning future care; it's also a legal record.

Formats used to document interventions include progress notes, flow sheets, and the medication administration record. In addition, you may use a special format for documenting emergency interventions. Alternative formats include the problem-oriented format, focus charting, and charting by exception.

Progress notes

Written in a traditional narrative (paragraph) format and in chronological order, progress notes include ongoing assessment data, nursing interventions, and patient responses.

How often should you document progress notes? The answer is determined by institutional policy in accordance with standards of your state and the Joint Commission on Accreditation of Healthcare Organizations. Because of recent efforts to decrease the amount of time that nurses devote to documentation, you should be aware of your facility's current policy. If you find that you're writing repetitious, meaningless notes, you may be charting too often.

Include in your notes changes in the patient's condition, new problems, the unchanged status or resolution of old problems, the patient's responses to treatments or medications, and the patient's or family members' responses to nursing interventions. Follow these guidelines when writing progress notes:
• Read the notes written by other members of the health care team before you write your own.

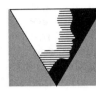

COLLABORATIVE PRACTICE

Strengthening cooperation between nurses and doctors

Institutional policy changes can have a profound effect on the level of cooperation between nurses and doctors. To initiate change, hospital administrators and staff need to honestly evaluate how doctors and nurses relate to each other. Do doctors communicate with nurses on a peer level? Do doctors and nurses recognize the role that nurses play in enhancing patient outcomes? Are nurses willing to accept responsibility and accountability for patient outcomes under their control? What position does the administration take when a conflict arises between a nurse and a doctor? Do doctors know and respect the organizational chain of command? Finding the answers to these questions will determine which policies and practices need to be changed to foster a collaborative approach to care.

The following policies are effective in fostering collaborative practice.

Integrated patient records
Interdisciplinary patient progress notes combine nursing and medical observations, judgments, and actions. They provide a formal means for nurses and doctors to communicate about patient care. These records also furnish a data base for monitoring implementation of joint standards and interdisciplinary quality assurance.

Joint practice committee
Staffed by nurses and doctors, a joint practice committee monitors professional cooperation and recommends action to support hospital-wide collaboration. Members of the health care team refer issues related to improving communication and efficiency to the committee. Doctors and nurses should receive equal representation and decision-making power and share responsibility for setting the committee agenda. Membership may be rotated periodically with meetings held monthly or bimonthly.

Joint review of patient care
Each month, a committee of nurses and doctors reviews patient charts to evaluate collaborative care. Joint review is particularly appropriate for specialty units, such as medical-surgical, critical care, and maternal-child health, in which specific groups of nurses and doctors interact closely and frequently.

Primary nursing
In primary nursing, one nurse is responsible and accountable for making decisions relating to continuous nursing care of a specific group of patients. Research indicates that primary nursing leads to greater patient and nurse satisfaction and better nurse-doctor collaboration. Direct and frequent contact between the same primary nurse

Strengthening cooperation between nurses and doctors — *continued*

and doctor during daily patient rounds strengthens communication and trust. The nurse is better able to exchange information and advocate a nursing plan of care that can be integrated with the medical care.

Independent clinical decision making by nurses

Policies and procedures should encourage each nurse to initiate care based on her independent judgment. Unit-specific protocols and standing orders can be used to clarify appropriate actions in situations where nurses must implement medical interventions (for example, emergencies). Remember that confusion and ineffective communication are less likely when medical and nursing roles are well defined.

Continuing education

A strong educational program fosters competence among nursing staff. Nursing knowledge and skills are the foundations for successful collaborative interventions. Collaborative responses from doctors are more likely if they trust the competence of the nursing staff.

• Read the notes recorded by nurses on other shifts, and make further comments on their findings to demonstrate continuity of care.
• If policy permits, use flow sheets to document repetitious procedures or measurements and summarize the information in the progress notes.
• Be sure to include specific information when you observe a change or lack of progress in your patient's condition, a response to treatment or medication, or a response to patient teaching.

Before you write your progress notes, organize your thoughts so that your paragraphs will be coherent. Use the patient's plan of care to review unresolved problems, expected outcomes, and prescribed interventions; then comment on the patient's progress based on these items. Discuss each problem in a separate paragraph; don't lump them together.

Progress notes require minimal training to use and understand and present a complete account of the care rendered and the patient's response; however, they can be tedious and lengthy. Also, organization and structure, accuracy, clarity, and style may vary, depending on each nurse's documentation skills.

Flow sheets

These abbreviated progress notes are used to document routine care measures, such as activities of daily living, wound care, vital signs, and other basic assessments. In many facilities, you may also use flow sheets to document I.V. monitoring, equipment checks, patient education, and discharge summaries. (See *Using a flow sheet for routine care.*)

Various flow sheet formats exist. Some are simple patient care checklists, others provide space for you to record specific care given, and some provide more space for evaluation statements.

Flow sheets are concise, legible, and accurate; therefore, they make documenting and reviewing documented material quick and easy. Specifically, they allow you to evaluate patient trends at a glance. But keep in mind that relying too heavily on flow sheets may fragment the documentation record, thereby obscuring the patient's clinical picture.

Medication administration record

The medication administration record (MAR) is a central document for recording medication orders and documenting their administration. Additional information, such as a patient's allergies to foods and medications, is also included in this document. The MAR is commonly contained in a Kardex file or on a separate medication administration sheet. When using an MAR, keep these guidelines in mind:
• Know and follow your facility's policies and procedures for recording medication orders and charting medication administration.
• Make sure that all medication orders include the patient's full name, the date, the name of the drug, and the dose, administration route or method, and frequency. Also make sure that the time of a stat dose is indicated. When appropriate, include the specific number of doses or the stop date.
• Write legibly.
• Use only standard abbreviations and use them correctly. When in doubt as to how to abbreviate a term, spell it out.
• After administering the first dose, sign your full name, licensure status, and initials in the appropriate space.

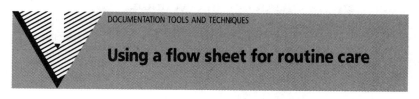

DOCUMENTATION TOOLS AND TECHNIQUES

Using a flow sheet for routine care

As this portion of a form shows, you can use a flow sheet to document routine interventions quickly.

PATIENT CARE FLOW SHEET

Date 1/22/94	11 p.m. to 7 a.m.	7 a.m. to 3 p.m.	3 p.m. to 11 p.m.
RESPIRATORY STATUS			
Lung sounds	CLEAR 12 AG	Crackles (R) ANT #9 chest BAL	Clear 4:30 BB 10 BB
Treatments & results	—	Nebulizer 10:30+ BAL	—
Cough & results	ō AG	Lg. amount 1030 Thick white mucus BAL	sm amount Thin, clear mucus 7:30 BB
O₂ therapy can 2 ℓ/m	continuous AG	with activity 12 BAL Pulse 90	with activity 7 BB pulse 92
CARDIAC STATUS			
Chest pain	ō AG	ō BAL	ō BB
Heart sounds	NORMAL S₁ AND S₂ AG	Normal heart sounds BAL	normal S₁ and S₂ BB
Telemetry	N/A	N/A	N/A
PAIN			
Type & location	SL. ABDOMINAL 2 AG	Abdominal 10 BAL	abdominal 7:30 BB
Intervention	VOIDED AG	Percocet, repositioning BAL	Tylenol — back rub BB
Response	IMMEDIATE IMPROVEMENT AG	Improved from #8 to #3	Complete relief in 1 hr BB
NUTRITION			
Type	—	Regular	Regular
Tolerance (%)	—	100%	50%
Supplement	—	— BAL	Soup from home BB
ELIMINATION			
Stool appearance	ō AG	↑ Light brown" BAL	ō BB
Enema & results	N/A	N/A	N/A
Bowel sounds	PRESENT 12 AG	Present all quadrants BAL	Present 4:30 BB
Urine appearance	CLEAR AMBER 2 AG	Light yellow 1 BAL	Light yellow BB
Foley catheter care	N/A	N/A	N/A
Catheter irrigation	↓	↓	↓

Documenting emergency interventions

When documenting an emergency, such as a cardiac arrest, you may need to use a special format, such as a code record, to consolidate all data in one place. (See *Using a code record.*) Be sure to take the following steps:

• Be specific about times and interventions, including medications administered.

• Include the name of the doctor you contacted, when you contacted him, and what you told him.

• Indicate attempts to inform the patient's family or significant other of changes in the patient's situation.

Alternative formats

Several alternative systems have been developed for documenting interventions: the problem-oriented format, focus-charting format, and charting-by-exception format.

Problem-oriented format

The problem-oriented medical record (POMR) system, sometimes called the problem-oriented record (POR) system, provides an integrated documentation format based on identified patient problems. With the POMR system, you'll document your interventions on one set of patient progress notes shared by all members of the health care team. The POMR system consists of five components: data base, problem list, initial plan, progress notes, and discharge summary.

The data base includes initial assessment data, such as patient history, physical examination, and other information obtained from the patient and family members.

The problem list includes the patient's current problems in chronological order according to the date each was identified. Usually, nurses and doctors keep separate lists, with problems stated as either nursing or medical diagnoses.

The initial plan includes expected outcomes, plans for further data collection (if needed), and treatment and patient education goals for each problem identified.

Progress notes are narrative notes written by all members of the health care team, using the SOAPIE format. This form is where you will document your nursing interventions. (See *Components of the SOAPIE format,* pages 152 and 153.)

The discharge summary covers each problem on the list and notes whether or not it was resolved. Plans for addressing unresolved problems may also be included.

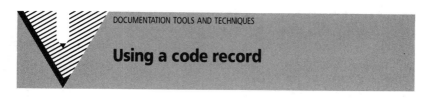

DOCUMENTATION TOOLS AND TECHNIQUES

Using a code record

This sample shows a portion of a code record, a special format used for documenting emergency interventions.

CODE RECORD

Name _Ray Walden_   Body weight _165lb_   Date _1/23/93_

Vital signs			Bolus meds						Infused meds			Actions			Blood gases			
Time a.m./p.m.	BP	Heart rate	Heart rhythm	Atropine (mg)	Calcium chloride (ampules)	Epinephrine (mg)	Lidocaine (mg)	Procainamide (mg)	Sodium bicarb (ampules)	Dopamine (mg/ml)	Isoproterenol (mg/ml)	Lidocaine (g/ml)	Defibrillation (joules)	CPR	Airway	PaO₂	PaCO₂	HCO₃	pH

Time a.m./p.m.	BP	Heart rate	Heart rhythm	Atropine	Calcium chloride	Epinephrine	Lidocaine	Procainamide	Sodium bicarb	Dopamine	Isoproterenol	Lidocaine	Defibrillation	CPR	Airway	PaO₂	PaCO₂	HCO₃	pH
8:20	0	0												✓	mask				
8:25	0	0	VF										200						
8:25														✓					
8:26													300						
8:27													360						
8:29						1	75							✓	E.T. tube	27	76	14	7.10
8:30													360						
8:31									1					✓					
8:31			↓										360						
8:32			NSR																
8:32			NSR																
8:35	140/90	96	↓				75									43	26	23	7.46

Time   Actions

8:20   Code called. CPR initiated by E. Land, RN, and J. Prince, RN
8:20   Bagged by J. Prince, RN
8:25   Single-channel ECG. Central line inserted via ® subclavian by Dr. Kee
8:29   ABG via ® femoral artery by Dr. Jay. Oral intubation by anesthesiologist.
8:32   Converted to NSR.
8:35   ABG via ® femoral artery. Pressure applied. Unresponsive.

Time code called _8:20_

Disposition

Status after resuscitation

☐ Arrest witnessed
☑ Arrest unwitnessed
☑ Intubation _8:29_
☑ Arrhythmia _V-Fib_
☑ Informed family

☐ SICU
☑ MICU
☐ CCU
☐ OR
☐ Morgue

_BP 140/90_
Heart rate 96. Bagged with
100% O₂ and transported
to MICU.

Components of the SOAPIE format

In the problem-oriented medical record system, all members of the health care team write narrative progress notes using the SOAP or SOAPIE format. If you use the SOAP format, you'll document the following information for each patient problem:

Subjective data: information that the patient and family members tell you

Objective data: factual data that you gather during physical assessment and from laboratory test results

Assessment: conclusions based on subjective and objective data that are formulated as patient problems or nursing diagnoses

Plan: your plan to relieve the patient's problems.

Some facilities use the SOAPIE format, adding:

Intervention: actions taken to achieve a patient outcome

Evaluation: an analysis of the effectiveness of your interventions.

You can easily adapt the SOAPIE format to your nursing diagnosis. Typically, you must write a SOAPIE note every 24 hours on any unresolved problem or whenever the patient's condition changes. You don't need to write an entry for each SOAPIE component; just omit the letter from the note or leave a blank space after it if you don't have any information to record, according to your facility's policy.

S
O
A
P
I
E

The POMR system's integrated documentation record enhances interdisciplinary communication, coordination, and continuity of care. It also unifies the plan of care and progress notes into a complete record of care. However, because information is buried in daily narrative notes, analyzing trends using this format is difficult. Also, documentation of interventions can become repetitious.

Focus-charting format
With this refinement of the SOAPIE format, you'll organize your thoughts into patient-centered topics, or foci of concern, and then document the foci precisely and concisely. Focus charting features columns for the date, time, focus, and progress notes.

With focus charting, first identify foci by reviewing the assessment data. Then write each focus as a nursing diagnosis,

Patient states that right arm is "heavy and clumsy." Reports to having "spells" of being unable to move right hand or arm, which feels numb and tingling. Having difficulty finding appropriate words. Episodes started 8 months ago, now occur every other day and last 10 minutes. Pt. has hypertension.

T, 98.8°F; P, 78 and regular; R, 22 and even and unlabored; BP, 182/96. Alert and oriented. Remote and recent memory intact. Speech slightly slurred. Pupils round, equal and reactive to light. Motor: right-handed. Upper and lower extremities strong bilaterally; right grasp weaker than left.

Knowledge deficit related to warning signs of stroke and importance of adhering to antihypertensive regimen. Correlates hypertension medications with feeling bad and having headaches.

Teach patient importance of following antihypertensive regimen and the warning signals of TIAs. Encourage patient to keep appointments.

Taught patient about antihypertensive regimen and importance of adherence. Explained TIAs and associated warning signs that should be reported. Gave patient printed material for reinforcement. Discussed importance of regular checkups to monitor blood pressure and TIAs.

Patient repeats some information and states that he will make a follow-up appointment.

a sign or symptom (for example, hypertension), a patient behavior or special need (such as discharge needs), an acute change in the patient's condition (such as loss of consciousness), or a significant event (such as surgery).

In the progress notes column, organize information using three categories: data, action, and response. In the data category, include subjective and objective information that describes the focus. The action category is where you'll document your nursing interventions. You should include immediate and future nursing actions based on your assessment of the situation as well as any changes to the plan of care that you deem necessary, based on your evaluation. Under the response category, describe the patient's response to any aspect of nursing or medical care.

By keeping the focus statement separate from the body of the progress notes, focus charting makes it easy to find information on a particular problem, thus facilitating communication among members of the health care team. It also highlights documentation of daily patient care and encourages regular recording of patient responses to nursing and medical interventions.

Charting-by-exception format

This format, probably the most abbreviated system, radically departs from traditional charting systems by requiring documentation of only significant or abnormal findings. It also uses military time to help prevent misinterpretations.

The charting-by-exception (CBE) format uses printed guidelines, such as nursing diagnoses–based standardized plans of care and protocols, in conjunction with several types of flow sheets, including the nursing-medical order flow sheet and graphic record.

The nursing-medical order flow sheet is used to document interventions. Each flow sheet is designed for a 24-hour period for one patient. (See *Using a nursing-medical order flow sheet.*)

The top of the form contains the orders for interventions. Each nursing order includes the corresponding nursing diagnosis number, labeled ND 1, ND 2, and so on; medical orders are identified by the initials "DO" (doctor's orders).

To document your interventions, use a check mark to indicate a completed intervention and an expected patient response. Indicate significant findings or abnormal patient responses with an asterisk, and write an explanation in the comments section. When the patient's response is unchanged, use an arrow.

The graphic record flow sheet is used to document trends in the patient's vital signs, weight, intake and output, appetite, and activity level. (See *Using a graphic record*, page 156.) As with the nursing-medical order flow sheet, use checks and asterisks to indicate expected and abnormal findings, respectively. Note information on abnormalities in the nurses' progress notes or on the nursing-medical order flow sheet.

In the box labeled routine standards, insert check marks to indicate that you've carried out established nursing care interventions, such as providing hygiene. You don't need to rewrite these standards as orders on the nursing-medical order flow sheet. Guidelines on the back of the graphic record usually provide complete instructions.

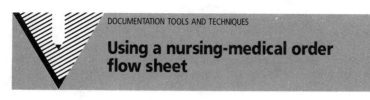

DOCUMENTATION TOOLS AND TECHNIQUES

Using a nursing-medical order flow sheet

This sample shows the typical features of a nursing-medical order flow sheet.

NURSING-MEDICAL ORDER FLOW SHEET

Patient's name __Linda D'Alessio__   Date __1/22/94__

ND# or DO	Assessment and interventions							
NDI	Integumentary assessment	1000 *	1100 *					
NDI	Vascular assessment	1000 ✓	1100 →					
ND2	Pain/comfort measure	1000 *	1100 *					
DO	Discontinue peripheral I.V.	1230 ✓						
Initials		DW	DW					

Key
DO = doctor's orders   → = no change in condition
ND = nursing diagnosis   * = abnormal or significant
✓ = normal findings   finding (see Comments
                                              below)

ND# or DO	Time	Comments	Initials
NDI	1000	Ⓛ Lower leg wound dressing saturated with pink-yellow nonodorous drainage. Re-dressed. Will reassess q 1 hr. ————	DW
ND2	1000	Pt. reports pain in Ⓛ lower leg at 8 on a scale of 1 to 10. Administered Percocet.—	DW
NDI	1100	No drainage on Ⓛ lower leg dressing.	DW
ND2	1100	Pt. reports pain improved to a 3. ——	DW

Initials	Signature
DW	Dorothy Wells, RN

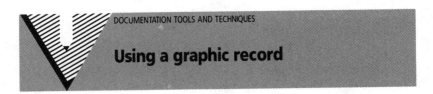

DOCUMENTATION TOOLS AND TECHNIQUES

Using a graphic record

This partial form illustrates how to use a typical graphic record.

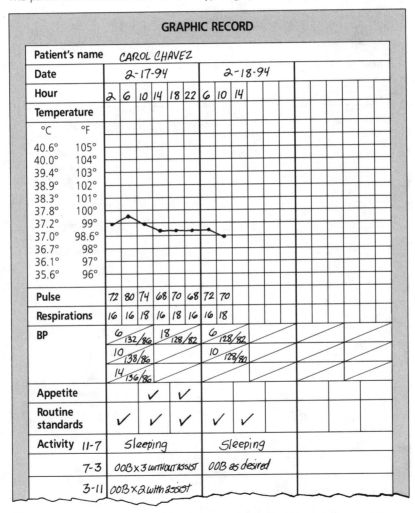

GRAPHIC RECORD

Patient's name	CAROL CHAVEZ																		
Date	2-17-94						2-18-94												
Hour	2	6	10	14	18	22	6	10	14										

Temperature

°C	°F
40.6°	105°
40.0°	104°
39.4°	103°
38.9°	102°
38.3°	101°
37.8°	100°
37.2°	99°
37.0°	98.6°
36.7°	98°
36.1°	97°
35.6°	96°

Pulse	72	80	74	68	70	68	72	70							
Respirations	16	16	18	16	18	16	16	18							

BP	6/132/86 18/128/82 10/138/86 14/136/86	6/128/82 10/128/80				

Appetite		✓	✓						
Routine standards	✓	✓	✓	✓	✓				

Activity 11-7	Sleeping	Sleeping
7-3	OOB x 3 WITHOUT ASSIST	OOB as desired
3-11	OOB x 2 with assist	

Because of its minimal narrative, the CBE format decreases the amount of documentation needed, eliminates redundant charting, and clearly identifies abnormal data. Plus, the flow sheets allow you to track patient trends easily. The CBE format also encourages you to document while providing bedside care. Its chief drawbacks are the major time commitment needed to develop clear protocols and standards of care and the extensive training required for the nursing staff and other members of the health care team. This radically different approach to documentation takes time to learn, accept, and use correctly.

KEY POINTS

• During implementation, the fourth phase of the nursing process, you put your plan of care into action. You use nursing interventions designed to achieve expected outcomes that have been agreed on by you and your patient.
• Interventions may be independent (initiated and carried out by a nurse), dependent (initiated by a doctor or other member of the health care team and carried out by a nurse), or interdependent (formed jointly by members of the health care team but carried out by a nurse).
• Examples of nursing interventions include assessing and monitoring the patient, providing therapeutic care, promoting comfort and function, supporting respiration and elimination, providing skin care, managing the environment, providing food and fluids, giving emotional support, teaching and counseling, and providing referrals to appropriate agencies and services.
• When you intervene, be sure that you understand the rationale for providing each intervention as well as possible adverse effects. Also, perform periodic reassessments, identify skills and knowledge that you'll need to perform nursing interventions, encourage family members to participate in the patient's care, and seek ways to increase your professional effectiveness.
• You can increase your professional effectiveness by improving your time-management skills and enhancing communication with colleagues.
• Five techniques can be used to resolve conflict: competition, accommodation, avoidance, compromise, and collaboration.

Usually, compromise and collaboration are the most effective strategies.

• You can foster collaboration between nurses and doctors in a number of ways. For instance, you can assess the relationships between doctors and nurses in your facility, encourage the implementation of integrated patient records, suggest the establishment of a joint practice committee, and recommend the implementation of joint review of patient care. You can also advocate the implementation of primary nursing, support the implementation of policies and procedures that provide a framework for independent clinical decision making by nurses, and promote the development of a strong educational program to foster competence among nurses.

• Formats used in documenting nursing interventions include progress notes, flow sheets, and the medication administration record. Alternative formats include the problem-oriented format, focus-charting format, and charting-by-exception format. You may also use a special format for documenting emergency care.

SELF-TEST

1. Assessing a patient's financial and insurance status to determine if he meets eligibility requirements for receiving aid from government or community resources is an example of which type of nursing intervention?

   a. physiologic
   b. psychological
   c. socioeconomic
   d. none of the above; this is not an appropriate nursing activity

2. When seeking to improve time-management skills, you should do all of the following *except:*

   a. plan your shift activities in advance.
   b. respond immediately to each patient request.
   c. learn to delegate.
   d. care for yourself as well as your patients.

3. When seeking to act assertively and confidently without appearing aggressive, you should do all of the following *except:*

a. state what you mean.
b. be mindful of your body language.
c. answer praise with such phrases as "Oh, it was nothing."
d. listen attentively.

4. When seeking to criticize a colleague in a constructive manner, you should do all of the following *except:*

   a. object only to actions the other person can change.
   b. present your criticism as a suggestion or question.
   c. voice your criticism as soon as possible.
   d. begin with a mild apology.

5. Which technique for resolving conflicts involves both parties modifying their behaviors to solve a problem?

   a. collaboration
   b. competition
   c. accommodation
   d. compromise

6. Which of the following is *not* an effective strategy for enhancing nurse-doctor collaboration?

   a. establishing a joint practice committee
   b. implementing integrated patient records
   c. promoting restricted accountability for nurses
   d. implementing primary nursing

7. When documenting the implementation phase, you should record:

   a. nursing observations and interventions.
   b. the times nursing interventions are performed.
   c. patient responses to treatments.
   d. all of the above.

8. A disadvantage of narrative progress notes is that they:

   a. tend to be tedious and lengthy.
   b. require extensive training to document correctly.
   c. are difficult to interpret.
   d. render only a partial account of nursing care delivered.

9. Which of the following would be considered the main disadvantage of relying too heavily on flow sheets to document your nursing interventions?

a. Flow sheets that become too long are difficult to read.
b. Flow sheets may fragment the documentation record.
c. Documenting information on flow sheets is tedious.
d. Documenting information on flow sheets is too time-consuming.

10. If you make the effort to research and find an appropriate support group for your patient and he refuses to attend, the most appropriate response would be for you to:

a. accept his refusal and go on to help other patients who are more willing to help themselves.
b. tell the patient he is in denial and needs counseling with a mental health professional.
c. assess whether the patient can help himself without the support group or if he is just denying his problems and feelings.
d. enlist family members and friends to encourage the patient to attend the group.

(Answers along with rationales can be found on page 262.)

FURTHER READINGS

Atkinson, L.D., and Murray, M.E. *Understanding the Nursing Process: Fundamentals of Care Planning,* 4th ed. New York: Pergamon Press, 1990.

Baugh, C. "Practical Ways to Assert Yourself," *Nursing89* 19(3):57, March 1989.

Better Documentation. Clinical Skillbuilders Series. Springhouse, Pa.: Springhouse Corp., 1992.

Bulechek, G.M., and McCloskey, J.C., eds. *Nursing Interventions: Essential Nursing Treatments,* 2nd ed. Philadelphia: W.B. Saunders Co., 1992.

Burke, L., and Murphy, J. *Charting by Exception.* New York: John Wiley & Sons, 1988.

Chouvardas, C.J. "Seven Steps to Asserting Yourself," *Nursing91* 19(3):126-32, November 1991.

Fayram, E.S. "Implementation," in *Nursing Process: Application of Theories, Frameworks, and Models,* 3rd ed. Edited by Christensen, P.J., and Kenney, J.W. St. Louis: Mosby-Year Book, Inc., 1990.

Fischbach, F.T. *Documenting Care: Communication, the Nursing Process and Documentation Standards.* Philadelphia: F.A. Davis Co., 1991.

Iyer, P.W., et al. *Nursing Process and Nursing Diagnosis,* 2nd ed. Philadelphia: W.B. Saunders Co., 1991.

Kuhn, R. "Nurse and Physician Collaboration: How to Strengthen the Team," *Heart and Lung* 14(5):18A, 20A, 21A, September 1985.

Lampe, S.S. "Focus Charting: Streamlining Documentation," *Nursing Management* 16(7):43-46, July 1985.

Lynch, M. "P-A-C-E Yourself: Tips on Time Management," *Nursing91* 21(3):104-08, March 1991.

McCloskey, J.C., et al. "Classification of Nursing Interventions," *Journal of Professional Nursing* 6(3):151-57, May-June 1990.

McFarland, G.K., and McFarlane, E.A. *Nursing Diagnosis & Intervention: Planning for Patient Care.* St. Louis: Mosby-Year Book, Inc., 1989.

Morgan, A.P., and McCann, J.M. "Nurse-Physician Relationships: The Ongoing Conflict," *Nursing Administration Quarterly* 7(4):1-7, Summer 1983.

Murphy, E.C. "Nurse-Physician Relationships: Part 2. Managing the Problem Relationship," *Nursing Management* 14(9):46-50, September 1983.

"On the Job: How to Deal with Criticism," *Nursing90* 20(2):123-24, February 1990.

"On the Job: Tips on How to Criticize," *Nursing91* 21(11):152, November 1991.

Pinnell, N.N., and de Meneses, M. *The Nursing Process: Theory, Application, and Related Processes.* East Norwalk, Conn.: Appleton & Lange, 1986.

Raudsepp, E. "Seven Ways to Cure Communication Breakdowns," *Nursing90* 20(4):132-42, April 1990.

Todd, S.S. "Coping with Conflict," *Nursing89* 19(10):100-09, October 1989.

EVALUATION

During evaluation, the last step of the nursing process, you judge the effectiveness of nursing care and gauge your patient's progress toward meeting expected outcomes. Evaluating the patient gives you the chance to:
• determine if original assessment findings still apply
• uncover complications
• analyze patterns or trends in your patient's care and responses to care
• assess his response to all aspects of care, including medications, changes in diet or activity, procedures, unusual incidents or problems, and patient teaching
• determine how closely care conforms with established standards
• measure the effectiveness of your care
• assess the performance of other health care team members
• discover opportunities to improve the quality of care.

The success of your evaluation depends largely on the quality of your plan of care. If you've clarified the plan's purpose and established measurable outcomes, you should have no trouble completing a thorough evaluation.

This chapter begins with an overview of the different types of evaluation. It divides evaluation into a series of simple steps and poses questions that you'll want to consider when evaluating reassessment data. The chapter also shows you how to write the evaluation (or patient outcome) statement—a documentation technique crucial to substantiating the rationales for your nursing care.

UNDERSTANDING TYPES OF EVALUATION

A *concurrent evaluation* takes place while your patient is still receiving care. In a formal evaluation, you use criteria established in your plan of care to evaluate your patient on an ongoing basis until he attains expected outcomes. In an informal evaluation, you don't define evaluation criteria but still review the patient's response to nursing care and make appropriate observations.

A *retrospective evaluation* occurs after contact with the patient has ended. By looking at patient outcomes, a retrospective evaluation seeks to monitor the quality and efficiency of care given. Tools used to conduct retrospective evaluations include closed-chart audits (such as reviews of nursing records), post-care patient interviews and staff conferences, and patient questionnaires.

Evaluation also may be objective, subjective, or a combination. *Objective evaluation* is based on data that you can observe and verify, such as the patient's vital signs. *Subjective evaluation* relies on your own perceptions and on the patient's verbal and behavioral responses to care. A subjective evaluation may also take into account information from secondary sources.

The most thorough evaluation combines subjective and objective methods. A combination approach helps to guard against the rigidity of an objective evaluation and the vagueness of a subjective evaluation and allows you to check for error by comparing results.

Both subjective and objective evaluations serve a purpose beyond assessing the individual patient. Data gathered from objective and subjective evaluations can be used to identify areas of future research as well as opportunities for improving care.

HOW EVALUATION PROCEEDS
An ongoing activity, evaluation usually overlaps with other phases of the nursing process. Your evaluation findings, in fact, may trigger a new cycle of assessment, nursing diagnosis, planning, implementation, and further evaluation. You may also uncover new information that will help you implement the plan of care more effectively.

To ensure a successful evaluation, keep an open mind. Never hesitate to consider new patient data or to revise previous judgments. After all, no plan of care is perfect. In fact, you should anticipate revising the plan of care sometime during the course of treatment. Keep in mind always that the patient's expected outcomes — the desired effects of nursing interventions — form the basis of evaluation. (See *Using an evaluation flowchart*, page 164.)

In the following section, you'll find the evaluation process divided into a series of steps: gathering reassessment data,

Using an evaluation flowchart

You can use the flowchart below as a guide throughout the evaluation process.

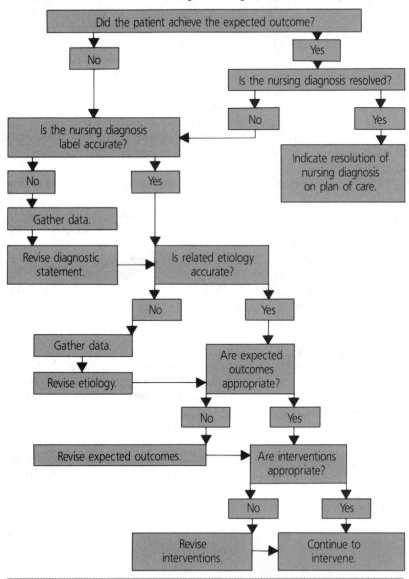

comparing reassessment findings with expected outcomes, identifying factors that interfere with goal achievement, writing evaluation statements, and revising the plan of care.

Gathering reassessment data

Reassessing the patient's status forms a crucial part of your evaluation. Techniques for gathering data include interviewing the patient, observing him, performing a physical examination, and reviewing the medical record.

How often should you reassess your patient? The answer hinges on his condition, but keep in mind that your institution and the Joint Commission on Accreditation of Healthcare Organizations (JCAHO) may stipulate a minimum frequency. If your reassessment uncovers new problems, you must revise the plan of care accordingly. (See *Revising nursing diagnoses*, page 166.)

Planned reassessment

During a planned reassessment, you collect routine data needed to evaluate the patient on a daily basis. Such data may include vital signs, 24-hour fluid status, self-care abilities, skin integrity, appetite, and respiratory, psychosocial, and mental status. Other factors to reassess regularly include environmental factors, learning needs, and discharge planning needs. Follow the reassessment parameters specified in your health care facility's unit-based performance standards. Based on the patient's condition, your plan of care may specify other reassessments as well.

Unplanned reassessment

Also called a documented reassessment, an unplanned reassessment may take place whenever a change occurs—for example, when the patient's status improves or deteriorates, when complications occur, when new therapies are initiated, when the patient undergoes invasive procedures or diagnostic tests, or when he receives a pass to participate in off-unit activities.

For example, suppose a patient with no previous cardiac dysfunction suddenly develops chest pain. You'd perform a complete assessment and schedule future cardiac reassessments according to the revised plan of care.

Or suppose you're caring for an elderly patient whose wife is his primary home caregiver. If his wife suddenly becomes incapacitated, you'd need to perform an unplanned reassessment of the patient's discharge needs.

Revising nursing diagnoses

In this case study, you'll learn how ongoing evaluation can reveal new patient problems. These problems, in turn, require development of new nursing diagnoses.

Cardiac complications

William Doran, age 76, is admitted to the hospital with cardiac arrhythmias. During the next few days, he has several episodes of chest pain that is relieved within 5 minutes by sublingual nitroglycerin. His vital signs are stable, but telemetry monitoring shows runs of atrial fibrillation interspersed with long periods of normal sinus rhythm. He has a history of chronic obstructive pulmonary disease; however, he stopped smoking more than 7 years ago.

Initial nursing diagnoses

Based on admission assessment findings, Marisa Wingate, Mr. Doran's primary nurse, chooses *decreased cardiac output* and *impaired gas exchange* as the nursing diagnoses. However, several days after his admission, she becomes concerned by his increasing restlessness and agitation. During a routine assessment, she asks Mr. Doran about his sleep and rest pattern.

"To tell you the truth," says Mr. Doran, lowering his voice to a whisper, "I haven't had a decent night's sleep here yet. My roommate keeps the television on all night and snores like a horse. I don't think I've slept more than 4 hours in the last 3 days."

New problems pinpointed

Marisa realizes that Mr. Doran now has two previously undiagnosed problems. She adds the nursing diagnoses *sleep pattern disturbance* and *anxiety* to the plan of care. To resolve these diagnoses, she develops new interventions, including arranging to move Mr. Doran to a private room and contacting his doctor to suggest a mild sedative to promote much-needed sleep.

Partial reassessment

You may need to perform a partial reassessment, in which you reassess one or more selected body systems. Suppose, for instance, that you're caring for a patient with a nursing diagnosis of *impaired gas exchange*. The plan of care may require you to periodically reassess the patient's respiratory status.

Team reassessment

At facilities that use a case management system, members of the health care team meet periodically during the patient's stay to reassess and evaluate his progress toward achieving established goals. The team determines if discrepancies exist between expected outcomes and patient progress.

If discrepancies exist, the team uses a variance record to document their frequency and type. A variance refers to something that alters a planned course of therapy. It may concern a patient, a member of the health care team, or the health care facility or system. For example, if a patient develops a wound infection that alters the expected outcome, a patient variance is noted on the record. If a doctor forgets to discontinue I.V. therapy and this interrupts the plan of care, a practitioner variance is noted. If a patient's hospital stay is prolonged because the hospital couldn't provide physical therapy on a weekend, a system variance is noted. (See *Using a variance record*, page 168.) Information on the variance record is used to revise and update critical paths.

Comparing reassessment data with expected outcomes

To evaluate the effectiveness of care, compare reassessment data with criteria established in expected outcome statements. Depending on the documentation format used by your health care facility, your comparison may also take into account outcome standards defined in protocols, hospital policy manuals, or other sources. (See *Fundamental questions for evaluating care*, page 169.)

For example, a patient with the nursing diagnosis *ineffective breathing pattern* might have the following expected outcomes listed in the plan of care:
• The patient's respiratory rate remains within ± 5 of baseline.
• The patient reports feeling comfortable when breathing.
• He demonstrates diaphragmatic pursed-lip breathing.
For this patient, you'll want to ensure that reassessment includes the patient's current respiratory rate, statements the patient has made about his comfort level when breathing, and observations of his ability to demonstrate pursed-lip breathing.

Your analysis of reassessment data should enable you to determine whether the patient's condition has improved, deteriorated, or stayed the same and whether any new complications have developed. You should also be able to determine which expected outcomes have been met, which have been partially met, and which haven't been met.

Identifying factors that interfere with achieving outcomes

You may find that your patient has achieved all of the expected outcomes by the projected dates. Or you may discover that

Using a variance record

When the health care team periodically evaluates the patient's progress toward achieving established goals, a variance record such as the one shown below may be used to document any discrepancies between expectations and the patient's progress.

DATE AND TIME	ITEM NOT ACCOM- PLISHED	VARI- ANCE TYPE	REASON	PLAN (ACTION)	DATE RESOLVED, INITIALS
8/17/93 9AM	Preop delay	PR	Medical clearance	obtained medical clearance/ surgery ASAP	8/18/93 RW
9/5/93 3PM	Discharge	Pt	Temp. elevation	change antibiotic	9/8/93 NL

VARIANCE TYPE		ADDRESSOGRAPH
PT = Patient PR = Practitioner S = System		STEVENS, LAURA DR. WONG, RM 311 8/16/93 #50094
Patient's name Stevens, Laura	Doctor Wong	Advance directive Y OR N

Reprinted with permission from Jane Barton, RN; Linda Brost, RN, BSN; Michelle Harrison, RN; and Martha Shinbeckler, RN, BSN, ONC; Orthopedic Unit, Overlook Hospital, Summit, N.J.

Fundamental questions for evaluating care

To help evaluate the effectiveness of care, you'll need to ask some fundamental questions. Based on the work of Carolyn G. Smith Marker, these questions identify the fundamental elements to consider when evaluating the patient's response to care:
• Is the patient stable or unstable?
• Is the patient's condition improving or deteriorating?
• Is the patient moving toward achieving outcomes or away from achieving outcomes?
• Are complications absent or present?

some patient problems have been only partially resolved or have not been resolved at all; if so, your next task is to assess factors interfering with goal achievement. Consider all possible reasons that a patient may not be able to achieve a desired outcome, such as those listed below:
• The purpose and goals of the plan of care aren't clear.
• The expected outcomes aren't realistic in light of the patient's condition.
• The plan of care is based on incomplete assessment data.
• Nursing diagnoses are inaccurate.
• The nursing staff experienced conflicts with the patient or medical staff.
• Staff members didn't follow the plan of care.
• The patient failed to carry out activities outlined in the plan of care.
• The patient's condition changed.

Reviewing implementation of the plan of care
When trying to determine factors that are interfering with goal attainment, you'll want to take a close look at whether the plan of care was implemented appropriately.

For example, suppose you're caring for a patient with the nursing diagnosis *decreased cardiac output,* who now weighs 8 lb (3.6 kg) more than he did on admission. To find out why he has failed to achieve the expected outcome of "patient exhibits little or no edema or weight gain," you'd review the nursing interventions listed on the plan of care. You'd ask yourself such questions as: Was a low-sodium diet ordered and given? Was the patient taught to elevate his feet when out of bed? Did the patient carry out planned activities? Were medications administered on time? Finding out the answers to these questions would help you determine why the expected outcome hasn't been achieved.

Reviewing implementation gives you a chance to monitor your own performance as well as judge your patient's progress. As you evaluate your patient's response to nursing interventions, determine if you're performing the interventions appropriately. Consider the following questions:
• Do I need new skills or information to implement the plan of care effectively?
• Have my personal feelings interfered with my ability to care for the patient?
• Did the staff provide continuity of care? Did other staff nurses participate in carrying out steps of the plan of care?

Writing evaluation statements

You may write several evaluation statements to document the patient's response to care. These statements should indicate whether expected outcomes were achieved and list the evidence supporting your conclusion. The importance of clearly written evaluation statements cannot be overemphasized: Documented patient outcome statements are necessary to substantiate the rationales for nursing care and to justify the use of nursing resources. You'll record your evaluation statements in your progress notes or on the revised plan of care, according to your facility's documentation policy.

Writing clear, concise evaluation statements is easy if you wrote precise expected outcomes when documenting your plan of care; expected outcome statements provide a model for documenting the evaluation. (In some documentation formats, such as patient care protocols, outcome standards may be specified for you.)

When documenting outcomes, describe the patient's progress using active verbs, such as "demonstrate," "express," or "walk." Include criteria used to measure the patient's response to care, and describe the conditions under which the response occurred (or failed to occur). Write a separate evaluation statement for each patient response or behavior that you wish to describe. Don't forget to date the evaluation statement.

Evaluation statements may cover a variety of topics, as in the following examples:

• Response to medical therapies and nursing interventions
   — Patient reports achieving pain relief 30 minutes after receiving 10 mg morphine sulfate I.M.
   — Patient's skin appears pink and less dusky after 20 minutes of oxygen administration at 2 liters/minute by nasal cannula.
   — Patient expresses feelings about being placed on full liquid diet; states that he's "always hungry and wants real food."
   — Patient shows no evidence of aspiration pneumonia. Breath sounds remain clear bilaterally; fever, chills, purulent sputum, and rapid shallow respirations are absent.
   — Patient shows no evidence of skin breakdown, contractures, or other complications of impaired physical mobility.
• Response to education and counseling
   — Patient successfully demonstrates ability to self-administer subcutaneous insulin.
   — Patient states three benefits of aerobic exercise program.
   — After reading literature provided by nurse, patient communicates understanding of medical regimen, diet, medications, and activity restrictions.
   — Family members display competence in caring for patient through return demonstration.
   — In aftermath of suicide attempt, patient makes verbal commitment to nurse not to act upon suicidal thoughts.
• Tolerance of increased activity
   — Patient demonstrates ability to walk on treadmill for 20 minutes without becoming fatigued.
   — Patient's blood pressure, pulse rate, and respiratory rate remain within prescribed range (specify) during periods of increased activity.
• Ability to perform activities of daily living (information that may be especially important for discharge planning)
   — Patient demonstrates ability to feed self using assistive devices.
   — Patient and caregiver demonstrate skill in managing incontinence, including use of external catheter and incontinence aids.

Revising the plan of care

You'll want to make sure that findings made in the evaluation process are recorded in the plan of care. When expected outcomes have been achieved, make sure that this information is recorded. Revise other expected outcome statements as necessary. Determine which nursing interventions need to be revised or discontinued. Check for changes in the priorities of nursing diagnoses, and document new problems that warrant new diagnoses.

Your evaluation may show that a nursing diagnosis has been resolved. When this happens, document this finding and modify the plan of care accordingly. (See *Documenting resolution of a nursing diagnosis.*)

You may find that a nursing diagnosis is still unresolved, even after you've revised the expected outcomes and developed

Documenting resolution of a nursing diagnosis

If your evaluation reveals that a nursing diagnosis has been resolved, document this on the plan of care. On the standardized plan below, the nurse has written "E" to document that the patient has been evaluated and "R" to document that the nursing diagnosis *altered tissue perfusion related to blood loss* has been resolved.

DATE 3/19/93	NURSE'S SIGNATURE *Susan Engler, RN*

Nursing diagnosis   Altered tissue perfusion related to blood loss

Patient outcomes
The patient will maintain adequate tissue perfusion, as evidenced by:
• systolic blood pressure above 90 mm Hg
• heart rate of 60 to 90 beats/minute
• urine output of at least 30 ml/hour
• baseline mental status.

Nursing interventions
• Monitor and record patient's vital signs every 15 minutes until stable, then every 4 hours for 24 hours; if blood pressure is low or pulse is high, notify doctor.
• Monitor intake and output every shift.
• Perform guaiac test on all stools and vomitus.
• Replace fluid volume as ordered.
• Administer oxygen as ordered.
• Monitor laboratory values and report any abnormal values to doctor.
• Monitor for and report signs of shock.

Specify:	**Date and RN signature**
E = Evaluated	*E* 3/21/93 *S. Engler, RN*
R = Resolved	*R* 3/22/93 *S. Engler, RN*

new interventions. If this happens, you will need to check the accuracy of the nursing diagnosis. Review the diagnostic label and etiology to see if it still describes the patient's status or problem. Then compare the defining characteristics with the patient's current signs and symptoms. You may discover that a new or revised diagnosis is needed.

KEY POINTS

• During evaluation, the last step of the nursing process, you judge the effectiveness of nursing care and gauge your patient's progress toward meeting expected outcomes.

• A concurrent evaluation takes place while your patient is still receiving care. Using criteria established in your plan of care, you evaluate your patient on an ongoing basis until he attains expected outcomes.

• A retrospective evaluation occurs after contact with the patient has ended. By looking at patient outcomes, a retrospective evaluation seeks to monitor the quality and efficiency of care.

• Evaluation may be objective, subjective, or a combination. Objective evaluation is based on specific facts. Subjective evaluation relies on your own perceptions and on the patient's verbal and behavioral responses to care. The most thorough evaluation combines subjective and objective methods.

• The patient's expected outcomes — patient-focused goals written in the planning phase and documented in the plan of care — form the basis of evaluation.

• Ongoing assessment is a crucial part of the evaluation process. The frequency with which you should reassess a patient depends primarily on his condition. Other guidelines for when to reassess include standards established by the JCAHO and the policies of your health care facility.

• Evaluation takes into account several different steps, including gathering assessment data, comparing reassessment findings with expected outcomes, assessing factors that interfere with goal achievement, writing evaluation statements, and revising the plan of care.

• During a planned reassessment, you collect routine data needed to evaluate the patient on a daily basis. Follow the reassessment parameters specified in the unit-based performance standards at your health care facility. An unplanned reassessment may take place whenever a change occurs—for example, when the patient's status improves or deteriorates.

• Each evaluation statement should document the patient's response to care, indicate whether the goals of the plan of care were achieved, and list the evidence supporting your conclusion. Evaluation statements are necessary to substantiate the rationales for nursing care and to justify the use of nursing resources.

SELF-TEST

1. Evaluation may be defined as:
   a. the last step in the nursing process.
   b. an opportunity to make judgments about the quality and appropriateness of nursing care.
   c. a dynamic and ongoing process that overlaps with other phases of nursing care.
   d. all of the above.

2. Why is the evaluation statement so important?
   a. It's the only documentation technique for noting when a patient hasn't achieved expected outcomes.
   b. It substantiates the rationales for nursing care and justifies the use of nursing resources.
   c. It separates information about the patient's response to nursing interventions from information about his response to medical interventions.
   d. It helps you determine when nursing diagnoses need to be revised.

3. Objective evaluation is based on:
   a. the patient's thoughts and perceptions.
   b. your thoughts and perceptions.
   c. data you can observe and verify.
   d. all of the above.

4. Which is the most important determinant for reassessing a patient?
   a. the patient's condition
   b. doctor's orders
   c. institutional policies

d. guidelines of the Joint Commission on Accreditation of Healthcare Organizations

5. What is the purpose of a retrospective evaluation?

a. to encourage members of the health care team to step back and contemplate the quality of patient care
b. to determine if nursing diagnoses are accurate
c. to monitor the quality and efficiency of care
d. to assess the quality of care while the patient is still under treatment

6. A nursing diagnosis is resolved when:

a. the patient attains expected outcomes associated with the diagnosis.
b. it becomes clear that the patient will never be able to attain expected outcomes associated with the diagnosis.
c. additional outcomes and interventions are added.
d. none of the above.

7. When evaluating your patient, you must determine if:

a. expected outcomes have been achieved.
b. expected outcomes have been achieved by the target dates.
c. the plan of care must be modified.
d. all of the above.

8. If the patient fails to achieve an expected outcome, you should:

a. assess factors that interfere with goal achievement.
b. review implementation of the plan of care.
c. revise interventions, expected outcomes, or nursing diagnoses, as needed.
d. all of above.

9. Criteria used during evaluation are established during which step of the nursing process?

a. assessment
b. planning
c. implementation
d. evaluation

10. Which of the following provides the best example of a clearly written evaluation statement?

    a. Patient feels better.

    b. Patient shows a lack of appreciation for the health care team's efforts by complaining approximately every 15 minutes.

    c. Patient reports achieving pain relief 40 minutes after injection of meperidine hydrochloride 75 mg I.M.

    d. Patient consumes adequate fluids each day and expresses anger in an appropriate way.

(For answers with rationales, turn to page 263.)

FURTHER READINGS

Accreditation Manual for Hospitals, 2 vols. Oakbrook Terrace, Ill.: Joint Commission on Accreditation of Healthcare Organizations, 1993.

Better Documentation. Clinical Skillbuilders Series. Springhouse, Pa.: Springhouse Corp., 1992.

Fox, L., and Woods, P. "Nursing Process—Evaluation of Documentation," *Nursing Management* 22(1):57-58, January 1991.

Iyer, P. "New Trends in Charting," *Nursing91* 21(1):48-50, January 1991.

Iyer, P., et al. *Nursing Process and Nursing Diagnosis,* 2nd ed. Philadelphia: W.B. Saunders Co., 1991.

Miller, D. "Complying with Joint Commission on Nursing Standards: Practical Documentation Tools," *Journal of Healthcare Quality* 14(1):24-29, January-February 1992.

Patterson, C. "Standards of Patient Care: The Joint Commission Focus on Nursing Quality Assurance," *Nursing Clinics of North America* 23(3):625-38, September 1988.

Smith Marker, C. *Marker Standards Based Documentation System (M-DOC).* Severna Park, Md.: Marker Systems, 1992.

Wells, P., et al. "COAD (Clinical Outcome Assessment Documentation) Charting: Using the Quality Improvement Process to Meet the New JCAHO Nursing Standards," *Journal of Healthcare Quality* 14(2):34-37, March-April 1992.

PART 2

EXPLORING ADVANCED
TOPICS

DISCHARGE PLANNING

For many patients, leaving the hospital and adjusting to home or long-term care proves stressful or even overwhelming. Discharge planning, however, aims to make this transition safe and smooth and to ensure continuity of care. Such planning is crucial because United States health care policy provides hospitals with a financial incentive to shorten patient stays.

This chapter describes the steps of discharge planning using the nursing process. You'll find signs to look for when determining a patient's discharge planning needs, guidelines for assessing the patient's home environment, and tips for increasing the effectiveness of your teaching. You'll learn what to communicate to home caregivers to ensure the patient's safety and how to record your discharge planning activities.

Discharge planning involves varied tasks, including teaching, documenting, organizing resources, and collaborating with other health care professionals. The patient's need for emotional support remains the one constant throughout this process. As a result, your most important role is support person, counselor, and patient advocate.

WHO'S RESPONSIBLE?
Hospital policy usually determines who holds responsibility for discharge planning. In some hospitals, the social service department bears primary responsibility. In others, a designated discharge planner, who may be a nurse or another member of the health care team, has responsibility. In most hospitals, though, staff nurses assume responsibility for discharge planning for patients under their care, sometimes working with a continued care coordinator. Whoever bears responsibility for creating the discharge plan also bears responsibility for supervising its implementation.

At times, the patient may come under the care of a discharge planning team that includes doctors, nurses, social workers, physical therapists, psychiatrists, and others. (See *Orchestrating the patient's discharge.*) Even if you don't have pri-

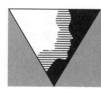

COLLABORATIVE PRACTICE

Orchestrating the patient's discharge

Successful discharge planning requires a multidisciplinary approach. The chart below describes the tasks of each member of the health care team.

Hospital administrator
Provides the necessary support to implement a discharge planning program

Staff nurse
Identifies patients who need continued care after discharge; assesses patient's mental status, functional abilities, and self-care deficits; assesses patient's home environment; determines discharge planning needs; collaborates with other health care team members in implementing a discharge plan; screens patients for home care referral; completes home health service request form; teaches patient and family members; provides written instructions to patient at discharge

Doctor
Establishes goals for patients; orders needed treatments before discharge; educates patient and family members on nature of the disease process, extent of disabilities, and necessary life-style changes; orders medications, treatments, equipment, and visiting nurse services; determines the need for follow-up appointments; communicates discharge plans to staff nurses, patient, and family

Psychiatrist
Evaluates patient's mental status; determines whether patient's competence is at issue and refers cases for court action, when necessary

Utilization review coordinator
Monitors utilization of hospital services; alerts discharge planning team when patients are medically ready to leave hospital

Social worker
Performs psychosocial assessment; evaluates patient's and family's strengths and weaknesses; counsels patient and family regarding concerns over illness or disability; assists with economic problems; assists patient in applying for Medicaid and other entitlement programs; refers patient and family to community resources; may be responsible for placing patient in long-term care facility

Physical, speech, and occupational therapists
Assess patient's functional abilities; set up rehabilitation programs; instruct family members in ways to assist patient; identify equipment needs

Orchestrating the patient's discharge—continued

Dietitian
Evaluates patient's dietary needs; teaches patient and family; arranges necessary supplies for enteral or parenteral nutrition

Community health nurse
Acts as liaison between hospital and home health care agency; collaborates with hospital staff nurse in formulating a plan of care based on medical history and nursing diagnoses; assesses patients for home health care needs; counsels patients and family members on the availability of home health care services; arranges for home health care; communicates patient information to home health care staff

---

mary responsibility for the discharge plan, you may play an important role as part of the discharge planning team. You and other team members will discuss the patient's discharge needs, propose appropriate plans, coordinate recommendations, and make sure that recommendations are implemented.

STEPS IN DISCHARGE PLANNING
Discharge planning should begin early during a patient's hospital stay. To ensure success, you'll need to accurately assess patient needs and encourage the patient and family members to participate as much as possible. The nursing process provides a good organizational framework for describing your responsibilities in discharge planning.

Assessment
The best time to explore a patient's discharge needs is during your initial assessment. Most hospitals have a standardized form for gathering assessment information. In addition to guiding inpatient care, assessment data can shape your plan for discharge.

If the patient's admission has been scheduled in advance, you may be able to begin discharge planning before the initial assessment. For example, if you know that the patient lives in a remote area with few services, he and his family will probably need detailed teaching and hands-on practice during hospitalization to master skills needed after discharge. In contrast, a patient who can rely on professional home health care may not need as much family training.

During assessment, try to anticipate the patient's condition at discharge. Will he likely have any self-care deficits? What will his functional mobility level be? Will he be able to perform activities of daily living, such as preparing meals and giving himself medication? Will he need skilled nursing care at home? Will he need full-time care in a facility?

Evaluate the patient's readiness to learn. Consider his mental and emotional state, how well he accepts his illness, and his level of motivation. Also assess family members' readiness to learn.

As you work through your assessment, be alert for signs that indicate the patient's specific discharge needs:
• special dietary needs or problems
• confusion about drug regimen
• noncompliance with drug regimen
• impaired ability to perform activities of daily living
• a need for treatments to be performed at home, such as I.V. therapy, wound care, tracheostomy care and suctioning, complex medication regimens, enteral feedings, colostomy or ileostomy care, or injections
• one or more functional disabilities
• urinary or bowel incontinence
• altered mental state
• insufficient social support
• limitations on physical activity
• signs and symptoms that need to be reported to the doctor
• questions or concerns about health
• a need for equipment to be used at home, such as oxygen or a walker.

Some hospitals use a screening form designed specifically for identifying discharge planning needs early in the patient's hospitalization (see *Using a discharge planning admission screen*, page 182).

Home environment
The patient's home environment can greatly affect his progress after discharge. To assess the home environment, ask questions such as:
• Does the home have a working telephone?
• Do stairs lead into the house? Are there stairs inside the house?

Using a discharge planning admission screen

A screening tool can be especially useful in determining a patient's discharge planning needs. To use the screening tool below, check off all indicators that signal a need for continued care after discharge.

Age and life-style indicators
☐ 70 or older
☐ Minor
☐ Transferred from other facility, such as a nursing home or a specialty hospital
☐ No known place of residence (homeless)
☐ Lives alone
☐ Coresident not capable of providing care

Symptomatic and behavioral indicators
☐ Noncompliant with plan of care
☐ Readmission within 31 days
☐ Attempted suicide or exhibits suicidal tendencies
☐ Possible or actual substance abuse
☐ Emotional or behavioral problems

Social and family indicators
☐ No identification carried by patient
☐ No family or social support system
☐ Family or domestic problems
☐ Overwhelming level of stress or fatigue for caregiver
☐ Single parent

Medical indicators
☐ History of forgetfulness or confusion
☐ Multiple trauma
☐ Head or spinal cord injury

☐ Physical disability, such as hearing or visual deficits or paralysis
☐ Psychiatric diagnosis or mental disability
☐ Chronic conditions or conditions that impair body function, such as chronic obstructive pulmonary disease, congestive heart failure, or cerebrovascular accident
☐ Suspected abuse or neglect
☐ Joint replacement
☐ Terminal illness
☐ Active communicable disease
☐ Taking multiple medications
☐ High-risk or complicated pregnancy
☐ Nutritional problems
☐ Ophthalmic procedure or condition

Nursing care and social service needs
☐ Needs follow-up care or referral to other agencies
☐ Limited financial resources or financial problems
☐ Currently uses a home health care agency
☐ Changes in body image (for example, amputation, burns, ostomy)
☐ Requires supportive services, such as shopping, transportation, housekeeping, laundry assistance, or Meals On Wheels
☐ Functional disabilities (specify)

• Does the patient require any special equipment that could prove difficult or hazardous in the house?

Find out who will help care for the patient when he returns home. How well do his friends and family function in supportive roles? These individuals greatly influence the patient's ability to function and recover at home.

Consider the capabilities of caregivers in addition to their availability and motivation. A weak, ill, or disabled family member may be unable to provide care no matter how willing he is to do so.

Keep in mind that most patients receive home care from their friends and family, not from professionals. If the patient does need professional home care, it should supplement, not replace, the care given by friends and family.

Nursing diagnosis

By providing a common language, nursing diagnoses can help you communicate a patient's postdischarge needs to other nurses in community agencies. This makes nursing diagnosis an excellent vehicle for discharge planning. Nursing diagnoses can help you pinpoint patient problems, including *impaired mobility, self-care deficit, knowledge deficit, social isolation, denial, anxiety, dysfunctional grieving,* or *urinary* or *bowel incontinence.* Using nursing diagnoses, you may be able to identify patient problems that other members of the health care team who are involved in the discharge process (such as administrators, doctors, therapists, and social workers) may overlook. In many health care facilities, you may be able to obtain patient care standards or protocols for selected nursing diagnoses that include postdischarge instructions.

Planning

Planning for discharge is an underlying element of the patient's entire hospital stay. Keep in mind that new needs and new nursing diagnoses may arise throughout the patient's hospitalization.

As you plan for the patient's discharge, take a holistic view of his needs. Consider his spiritual, cultural, and ethnic beliefs and his psychological response to illness and disability, as well as his physiologic needs. Family communication patterns, strengths, and weaknesses should also be considered. Take into account the patient's expressed wishes when developing the discharge plan. Encourage the patient and his family to participate in formulating the plan.

Think about the patient's anticipated length of stay, and plan ahead so that the patient and his family have time to learn what they need to master before discharge. Document the anticipated length of stay and the patient's learning needs on the nursing plan of care.

If appropriate, think about referring the patient or family members to a self-help group or another community resource. In many cases, a social worker will be available to help you in providing such referrals. This intervention requires careful consideration. Become familiar with the support groups in your community. Check to see if your hospital has a directory of community resources and support groups; consider visiting groups to which you'll probably refer patients.

Documenting the discharge plan

How you document the discharge plan will depend on the policy at your health care facility. Some policies require you to include your assessment of discharge needs on the initial assessment form, then document the discharge plan itself on a separate form. At many facilities, you must include the discharge plan as a component of the discharge summary. (The discharge summary is used to document patient status at the time of discharge, specific discharge instructions given, and the patient's or family's understanding of the instructions.) Discharge needs also may be documented in progress notes or in a flow sheet format. Some forms used for discharge planning allow several members of the health care team to include information.

Whatever format you use, the discharge plan should include the following information: nursing diagnoses, the patient's anticipated length of stay, the patient's learning needs, medications and treatments that must be continued after discharge, diet instructions, physical activity limitations, signs and symptoms that the patient or caregiver should report to the doctor, follow-up medical care needs, equipment needs, available assistance, and appropriate community resources and support groups.

Implementation

Interventions may include teaching the patient and caregivers, arranging for outside services, conveying instructions to the staff of a home health care agency or long-term care facility, introducing the patient to self-help groups or other community resources, and providing the patient with written instructions that he can follow after discharge.

Teaching the patient and family
Teaching may be as simple as explaining the need for a follow-up medical appointment or as complex as teaching family members how to care for an incontinent patient confined to bed who needs enteral feedings and suctioning.

Ideally, you'll develop a formal teaching plan, arrange a time to meet with the patient (and family members), and work together toward specific learning goals. In practice, you need to be flexible. The most important teaching may occur when the patient or a family member asks you questions when you're in the room for another reason.

• *Seize the moment.* Teaching is most effective when it occurs in quick response to a need the learner feels. So even when you're busy administering treatment for a pressure ulcer, make every effort to teach the patient when he asks, "What can I do to stop getting so many open sores?" Your formal teaching plan may be in the patient's chart or on your desk, but the patient is ready to learn now. Satisfy his immediate need for information, and augment your teaching with more information later.

• *Involve the patient in planning.* Just presenting information to the patient won't ensure learning or change. For learning to occur, you'll need to involve the patient in identifying his learning needs and expected outcomes. Help him to develop attainable outcomes.

• *Begin with what the patient knows.* You'll find that learning moves faster and easier when it builds on what the patient already knows. A patient who has been on peritoneal dialysis and is being changed to hemodialysis has some exposure to the concept of fluid exchange. To teach him, begin by comparing the old known process with the new unknown one. He'll be able to grasp the new information more quickly.

• *Move from the simple to the complex.* The patient will find learning more rewarding if he has the opportunity to master simple concepts first and then to apply these concepts to more complex problems. Keep in mind, however, that what one patient finds simple, another may find complex.

• *Use the patient's preferred learning style.* How quickly and well a patient learns depends not only on his intelligence and education but also on his preferred learning style. Visual learners gain knowledge best by seeing or reading the information; auditory learners, by listening; and tactile or psychomotor learners, by doing. You may also combine learning styles; lessons are most likely to be retained if the patient

reads, hears, and repeats information and performs associated skills.
• *Sort goals by learning domain.* Learning behaviors fall into three domains: cognitive, psychomotor, and affective. The cognitive domain deals with intellectual abilities. The psychomotor domain includes physical and motor skills. The affective domain involves expression of feelings, attitudes, interests, and values. Categorizing the patient's learning needs in the appropriate domain helps identify and evaluate the behaviors you expect him to exhibit.
• *Make material meaningful.* Another way to facilitate learning is to relate material to the patient's life-style and ways of thinking—and to recognize incompatibilities. For example, teaching a patient who's had a cerebrovascular accident how to prepare his own meals may be futile if he believes that his spouse ought to do all the cooking.
• *Allow immediate application of knowledge.* Giving the patient the opportunity to apply his new knowledge and skills reinforces learning and builds confidence. For example, providing a diabetic patient with sample menus and asking him to rehearse selecting meals may help reinforce teaching about diet and nutrition.
• *Tell the patient how he's progressing.* Learning is easier when the patient is aware of his progress. Positive feedback can motivate him to greater effort because it makes his goal seem attainable. Rather than simply offering general encouragement and praise, be sure to recognize specific behaviors. Praising desired behavior improves the chances of the patient repeating that behavior. Reassuring him that he has learned the technique can help him refine it and can motivate him to practice.

Documenting patient teaching
In the patient's medical record and in any home health referrals, document exactly what you taught and the patient's and family's response to that teaching. Document any return demonstration of skills performed by the patient or his family. Write clearly and provide complete explanations: Your notes provide a permanent legal record of the content of your teaching and the responses to it. (See *Outcome criteria for discharge planning.*)

Documentation saves time by preventing duplication of patient-teaching efforts by other staff members. By checking your notes, another nurse can determine what has been covered and what she should teach next, without skipping essen-

Outcome criteria for discharge planning

When teaching your patient the skills necessary to ensure a successful hospital discharge, you should devise outcomes that clearly state the behavior that the patient needs to learn. By basing your discharge plan on outcome criteria, you can better prepare the patient for the transition to home or long-term care facility. By checking off what he demonstrates he can do, you can document what the patient has actually learned.

The list below provides examples of outcome criteria that can help determine whether your patient is prepared for discharge.

Appointments
• Patient schedules appointment with his doctor or states when he should make an appointment.
• Patient states reasons for calling doctor or nurse before the scheduled appointment (for example, bleeding, swelling, increased pain, or other complications).

Diet
• Patient describes diet he must follow after discharge.
• Patient explains the rationale for his diet.
• Patient states whom to call with questions about his diet.
• Patient explains restrictions regarding fluid intake.

Medications
• For each medication he takes, patient states:
  – its name
  – the proper dose
  – how often he takes it
  – when he takes it (before or after meals)
  – why he takes it
  – special precautions and potential adverse effects
  – when to contact the doctor concerning the medication.

Treatments and procedures
• Patient or caregiver demonstrates ability to perform any necessary treatments, procedures, and dressing changes.
• Patient states where to obtain necessary equipment, supplies, and dressings.
• Patient explains how equipment is used during treatment or procedure.
• Patient explains how to dispose of soiled dressings.

(continued)

Outcome criteria for discharge planning — *continued*

Activity
• Patient states recommendations for increasing activity level (for example, increase walking to 1 mile within 3 weeks).
• Patient states limitations regarding positioning, weight bearing, lifting, and stair climbing.
• Patient demonstrates prescribed exercises.

Community resources
• Patient explains rationale for using home-care services.
• Patient lists community resources available to him (for example, American Cancer Society chapter, community task force on acquired immunodeficiency syndrome, stroke club, hot lines, and support groups).

---

tial information. This is especially important for patients with complicated needs who receive care from several nurses.

In many health care facilities, you'll document patient teaching on preprinted forms that become part of the clinical record. If your facility doesn't have a preprinted form, write accurate narrative notes.

Requesting home care services
If the patient will need services at home, expect to complete a home health services referral form as part of implementing the discharge plan. The format used to request home health services varies among hospitals, but the purpose is always the same: to provide the home health care agency with the information needed to care for the patient properly. You can help ensure a safe transition from hospital to home by providing complete, accurate information. (See *Using a home care referral form.*) Include the following information:
• patient's name, address, and phone number
• directions to the patient's home, including floor number, apartment number, or any other helpful notes
• an emergency contact
• patient's medical diagnosis
• medical history
• diet instructions
• activity level or restrictions
• an indication of why the doctor made the referral for home care

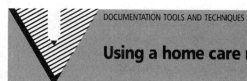

DOCUMENTATION TOOLS AND TECHNIQUES

Using a home care referral form

To make sure that the patient returns home safely, provide complete information on the home care referral form.

HOME HEALTH SERVICES REFERRAL

Recorded by _Cindy Flaherty_

Date _8/25/93_

Referral source/Dept. _4 North_

Patient _Frank Dupree_ _____ Telephone # _698-2121_

Address _343 Lawndale, Salt Lake City_ _____ Zip _84132_

Directions to home _West on 300 to Devon exit, right on Market._
2nd left is Lawndale

Emergency contact (name and telephone number) _Daniel Dupree (son)_
_745-0776_

Birth date _03-16-27_ Age _66_ ____ Marital status _Widower_

Medical diagnoses/surgical procedure _MI, Balloon angioplasty_

Nursing diagnoses _self care deficit, knowledge deficit, alteration in nutrition_

Medical history/hospitalizations _Cholecystectomy, 1987_
Pneumonia, 1989

Facility discharged from _University Hospital_ ____ Unit _____

Date of discharge _8/26/93_ _____ First home visit _8/31/93_

☑ Medicare # _543-12-3454_ ____ ☐ Medicaid # _____

☐ Insurance ID # _____

Insurance benefits to be reviewed with family _____

Medical orders/supplies _Outpatient cardiac rehab program, home followup c̄_
home health nurse, weekly BP and CBC, lytes. Stop smoking clinic.

Medications _Isordil, 20 mg TID, Vasotec 10 mg QD, Lasix 40 mg QD,_
enteric coated aspirin TQD

Doctor _Dr. K. Harrison_ _____ Telephone or beeper # _698-0103_

Baseline assessment

Height _5'8"_ ____ Weight _220 lbs_ T _98.6°F_ P _82_ ____ R _16_

BP, right arm _144/92_ ____ BP, left arm _140/88_

Nursing assessment/recommendations
Encourage patient to change living habits; monitor diet;
ask about attendance in stop smoking clinic

Comments
Patient needs to be made aware of relationship between
lifestyle and cardiac health

• nursing diagnoses and your assessment of the patient's needs
• a list of the patient's medications
• dates of the patient's admission and discharge
• which unit the patient was on while in the hospital
• supplies that the home care nurse will need to order
• patient's financial status (including such information as the number of home care visits authorized by the patient's insurance company)
• a brief nursing assessment of the patient, including mental status, psychosocial status, mobility, baseline vital signs, elimination patterns, skin condition, diet and appetite, and any self-care deficits
• specific treatments ordered.

Providing patient instructions

You'll probably need to provide the patient with written instructions when he leaves the hospital. Many hospitals have patient instruction forms for you to use. To make documentation quicker and easier, many facilities have developed combined discharge summary and patient instruction forms. (See *Using a discharge summary and patient instruction form.*) This documentation tool combines all the essential information required on a discharge summary as well as the instructions given to the patient. Ideally, you should fill out the discharge instruction form a day or two before discharge. Usually, you'll keep one copy of the form in the clinical record and give one copy to the patient at discharge. The copy you keep may be used for further teaching and evaluation.

The instruction sheet will reinforce your patient teaching and help the patient remember what to do. It may also list signs and symptoms to report to the doctor, the date of a follow-up appointment, and any contraindicated activities. Don't forget to include instructions about the drug regimen and potential adverse effects.

Do your best to adapt written instructions to your patient's special needs. For example, if your patient is illiterate, use pictures. If your patient does not read English, seek a translator who can copy the information into the patient's language.

Evaluation

You'll be evaluating the patient's discharge plan as his needs change during his hospital stay and after he is discharged from the hospital.

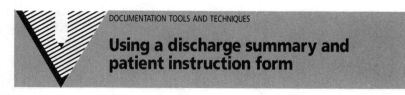

DOCUMENTATION TOOLS AND TECHNIQUES

Using a discharge summary and patient instruction form

This sample form combines your discharge summary with your postdischarge instructions for the patient. You'd give a copy of this form to the patient at discharge.

DISCHARGE SUMMARY

Date __1/25/94__

Time __2 p.m.__

Patient __Andrew Daymon__

Destination
- [x] Home
- [ ] Nursing home
- [ ] Other _____

Mobility
- [x] Ambulatory
- [ ] Wheelchair
- [ ] Stretcher

PATIENT STATUS
General
- [x] TPR __98.6° – 76 – 16__
- [x] BP __134/82__
- [ ] Eating regularly

Comments _____

Skin
- [x] Good condition
- [x] Wound __① Leg wound healing well__
- [ ] Other _____

Bowels
- [x] Regular movement
- [ ] Irregular movement
- [ ] Ostomy

Bladder
- [x] Continent
- [ ] Urinary frequency
- [ ] Incontinent
- [ ] Catheter

Type _____

Date changed _____

Compliance
- [x] Understands physical condition
- [x] Willing to comply with regimen
- [x] States understanding of instructions

Comments __Gave successful return demonstration of ① leg wound dressing change__

Medications
- [ ] Preadmission medications returned
- [x] Prescriptions given to patient
- [ ] Medications given to patient
- [x] Patient or family knows of allergies

Nurse's signature __Barbara A. Lane, RN__

(continued)

Using a discharge summary and patient instruction form – *continued*

PATIENT INSTRUCTIONS

Diet
- ☑ Unrestricted
- ☐ Restricted _____

Activities
- ☑ Walking
- ☑ Climbing stairs
- ☑ Riding in car
- ☑ Driving car
- ☑ Showering
- ☐ Taking a tub bath
- ☑ Engaging in sexual intercourse
- ☑ Resuming regular activity
- ☑ Lifting
- ☐ Exercising

Other _____
Comments *Avoid strenuous exercise until wound completely heals*

Medications (include dosage, route, and time)
Percocet, 1 tablet orally every 6 hours as needed for pain relief

Special instructions
_____
_____
_____
_____
_____
_____

Referral
- ☑ Call Dr. *Wilson*

and schedule an appointment for
2 weeks from today .
- ☐ Home care agency _____

Other _____

If you have questions, call Dr. *Wilson*
at *555-1937* .

I've read and understood these instructions, and I've received a copy of this form.

Date *1/25/94*

Patient's or significant other's signature

Janice Hart

Nurse's and doctor's signatures

Barbara A. Lane, RN

Dr. H. Wilson, MD

Before the patient leaves the hospital, ask yourself if he is really ready to go home. Think about whether all the needed arrangements have been made. And most important of all, if you think plans are inadequate or your patient is not prepared, speak out. Because of the pressure to discharge patients from the hospital quickly, you may have to act as a patient advocate to ensure that the patient receives the discharge services he needs.

Some hospitals have a designated staff member who is responsible for making follow-up phone calls to the patient after discharge. Home health care agencies may facilitate follow-up by calling the hospital to report on the patient's status.

Use the questions below when seeking to evaluate the effectiveness of discharge planning services and the success of the patient's transition from hospital to home or long-term care facility:
• Are equipment and support services in place for the patient's return home?
• Did the patient and family actively participate in forming the discharge plan?
• Does the discharge plan take into account the patient's spiritual and cultural practices, his physical and psychological responses to illness and disability, and family communication patterns and strengths and weaknesses?
• Are the nursing diagnoses in the discharge plan accurate?
• Did the patient and family receive all necessary instructions before leaving the hospital? Do they understand their home care instructions?
• Did the patient receive adequate emotional support during a difficult transition from hospital to home or long-term care facility?
• Are home health services adequate? Does the patient have access to skilled nursing care? Are home health aides carrying out provisions of the discharge plan?
• Is the patient making use of support groups or other recommended community resources?
• Do home care personnel have all the medical and psychosocial information needed to ensure continued quality of care?
• Is the patient following the prescribed diet and medication regimen at home? Are the patient and family using special equipment correctly?
• How has the patient's return home affected family coping? Do family members function effectively in the supportive role?
• Has immediate readmission after discharge been avoided?

• Usually, staff nurses are responsible for discharge planning, but this varies among hospitals. Whoever takes primary responsibility for developing the patient's discharge plan is also responsible for supervising its implementation.

• As the length of the average hospital stay decreases, the need for thorough discharge planning increases. The sicker the patient is when he leaves the hospital, the greater the need for postdischarge care.

• The best time to explore a patient's need for discharge planning is during your initial assessment. Most hospitals have a standardized form for gathering assessment information. In addition to guiding inpatient care, assessment data can tell you much about discharge planning needs.

• The patient's home environment can greatly affect his progress after discharge. Assess the home environment, paying close attention to the amount and quality of social support available to the patient. You should also consider the willingness and capability of family and friends to assist with care.

• Important techniques to ensure successful learning include seizing the moment when responding to the patient's learning needs, involving the patient in planning, beginning with material the patient knows, moving from the simple to the complex, using the patient's preferred learning style, sorting goals by learning domain, making material personally meaningful to the patient, providing an immediate opportunity for the patient to apply new knowledge, and making the patient aware of his progress.

• If the patient will need services at home, you'll have to complete a home health services referral form. The format used to request home health services varies among hospitals, but the purpose is always the same: to provide the home health care agency with the information needed to care for the patient properly.

• You'll probably need to provide the patient with written instructions when he leaves the hospital. These instructions should reinforce patient teaching and may include signs and symptoms to report to the doctor, the date of a follow-up appointment, any contraindicated activities, diet instructions, and instructions about the drug regimen and potential adverse effects.

1. In most cases, how would you determine who is responsible for discharge planning?

    a. Refer to hospital policy.
    b. Ask the patient which member of the health care team he trusts the most.
    c. Follow doctor's orders.
    d. Refer to state law.
    e. None of the above.

2. What is the main reason that discharge planning is becoming increasingly important?

    a. Patients have a greater awareness of their health care needs.
    b. The length of the average hospital stay is decreasing.
    c. Because of the breakdown in family structure, patients receive less support from family and friends.
    d. New regulations by the Joint Commission on Accreditation of Healthcare Organizations (JCAHO) require that hospitals provide a detailed account of each patient's discharge plans.

3. When should you begin evaluating a patient's need for post-discharge care?

    a. when he begins asking you questions about his condition
    b. when family members express a willingness to discuss his illness
    c. during your initial assessment
    d. after 48 hours
    e. on the day of discharge

4. The implementation phase of discharge planning may involve:

    a. referring your patient to a self-help group.
    b. providing written instructions for him to take home.
    c. teaching the patient and family home-care procedures.
    d. arranging for outside services.
    e. all of the above.

5. Most patients receive the bulk of their postdischarge home care from:

   a. home health care agencies.
   b. nurse's aides.
   c. community support groups.
   d. family and friends.
   e. registered nurses.

6. Which of the following is *not* a responsibility of the staff nurse in the discharge planning process?

   a. identifying patients who need continued care after discharge
   b. evaluating mental status to determine whether the patient's competence is at issue
   c. completing a home health service request form
   d. assessing the patient's home environment
   e. all of the above may be part of the staff nurse's responsibility, depending on hospital policy

7. If you wish to provide discharge instructions to a patient who is illiterate you should:

   a. encourage the patient to enroll in an adult literacy program.
   b. give written instructions to the patient's significant other.
   c. use pictures to communicate your instructions.
   d. write instructions using the phonetic alphabet.
   e. none of the above.

8. If the patient is about to leave the hospital and you feel he is not adequately prepared for discharge, you should:

   a. speak out to ensure the patient's safety and well-being.
   b. keep quiet to protect your health care facility from potential liability.
   c. refuse to sign the discharge summary.
   d. inform home care personnel that they must be especially careful.
   e. none of the above.

9. If you are in the middle of performing a nursing procedure and the patient interrupts with a question about his care, you should:
   a. adhere as closely as possible to the schedule outlined in your formal teaching plan.
   b. evaluate the patient's motives to see if he is actually expressing fear or anxiety.
   c. provide an answer to the patient's question and follow up with more information later.
   d. politely tell the patient that you'll return later to discuss his concerns.
   e. do any of the above; it depends on the situation.

10. Why do you perform an assessment of the patient's home environment as part of discharge planning?
   a. JCAHO standards require that discharge planning include an assessment of the home environment.
   b. The patient's home environment can greatly affect his progress after discharge.
   c. Increasing social problems, such as elder, spouse, and child abuse, have made an assessment of the home environment essential.
   d. You would not perform an assessment of the home environment as part of the discharge planning process.

(For answers with rationales, turn to page 264.)

FURTHER READINGS

Blaylock, A., and Cason, C.L. "Discharge Planning: Predicting Patient Needs," *Journal of Gerontological Nursing* 18(7):5-10, July 1992.

Chappell, H.W. "Nurses' Commitment Makes a Difference in Discharge Planning," *Kentucky Nurse* 37(3):13-14, May-June 1989.

Corkery, E. "Discharge Planning and Home Health Care: What Every Staff Nurse Should Know," *Orthopaedic Nursing* 8(6):18-27, November-December 1989.

Dumas, L. "How to Tie Up the Discharge Plan," *RN* 50(4):81-82, April 1987.

Edwards, J., et al. "An Analysis of the Quality and Effectiveness of the Discharge Planning Process," *Journal of Nursing Quality Assurance* 5(4):17-27, July 1991.

Foster, S.D. "The Role of Education in Discharge Planning," *MCN* 13(6):403, November-December, 1988.

Fritsch-deBruyn, R., and Cunningham, H. "A Check on Nurses' Knowledge and Sense of Responsibility for Discharge Planning," *Journal of Nursing Staff Development* 6(4):173-76, July-August, 1990.

Gilchrist, B. "Discharge Planning: A Priority for Nurses," Part 2. *Geriatric Nursing & Home Care* 7(12):16-18, December 1987.

Kerson, T.S. "Home-focused Discharge Planning," *Health and Social Work* 15(3):243-45, August 1990.

Knight, S. "Assessment to Discharge, This Form Does It All," *RN* 52(7):36-40, July 1989.

Mezzanotte, E.J. "A Checklist for Better Discharge Planning," *Nursing87* 17(10):55, October 1987.

Thliveris, M. "A Hospitalwide Discharge Planning Program," *Dimensions in Health Service* 67(1):38-39, February 1990.

Weinberger, B. "Discharge Planning: The Sooner, the Better," *Nursing89* 19(2):75-76, February 1989.

Wilson, E.B., et al. "Take a Fresh Look at Discharge Planning," *Geriatric Nurse (New York)* 12(1):23-25, January-February 1991.

LEGAL ISSUES

The nursing process has helped to establish nursing as a distinct profession with its own body of knowledge. As part of attaining greater professional recognition, nurses have had to accept stricter legal accountability. This accountability, in part, rests on established standards of care. For instance, standards are commonly incorporated into state nurse practice acts as well as hospital policies and protocols. Accepted national standards are becoming increasingly important in how courts rule on issues of nursing negligence or malpractice.

This chapter covers recent standards issued by the American Nurses' Association (ANA) and the Joint Commission on Accreditation of Healthcare Organizations (JCAHO). You'll learn what these two important organizations have to say about the nursing process and nursing diagnoses. You'll also learn exactly what you must do to practice in accordance with their standards.

Both the ANA and the JCAHO require that you document your use of the nursing process. In effect, your documentation records how well you've met standards of care. Because the law views nursing documentation seriously, the chapter includes a special section on the legal significance of nursing documentation and ways to avoid charting errors that can undermine your credibility in court.

STANDARDS OF CARE

Nursing care standards set minimum criteria for nursing proficiency. They describe the activities for which you're accountable. And they provide a direction for professional nursing practice and guidelines for evaluating practice. Becoming aware of professional nursing standards will help you judge the quality of care that you and your nursing colleagues provide.

Unless they're incorporated into your state's nurse practice act, professional standards aren't laws. Rather, they're guidelines for sound nursing practice. Nevertheless, to protect yourself legally, your care should meet the general standards described in this chapter. If you can't prove that your care meets accepted standards, you increase your risk of being held liable for negligence or malpractice. (See *Nursing standards and the courts.*)

Evolution of nursing standards

Before 1950, nurses had only Florence Nightingale's early treatment records, plus reports of court cases, to use as standards. In 1950, though, the ANA published the *Code of Ethics for Nursing.* This code states that nurses should provide care without prejudice and in a confidential and safe manner. Although nonspecific, the code marked the beginning of written nursing standards. In 1973, the ANA Congress for Nursing Practice established the first generic standards for the profession — standards that could be applied to all nurses in all settings.

Currently, the ANA and JCAHO are two of the most important organizations setting standards for nursing care. Some states have incorporated their standards into nurse practice acts. Your facility probably has integrated their standards into its own policy and procedure manual.

As technology advances and nursing responsibilities expand, nursing standards change as well. Both the ANA and the JCAHO continually monitor nursing standards to make sure that they're up to date. In 1991, the JCAHO revised its nursing care standards. That same year, the ANA published its revised *Standards of Clinical Nursing Practice.*

ANA standards

As the professional association for registered nurses in the United States, the ANA develops and publishes standards of care for the nursing profession. ANA standards are generic–they apply to all registered nurses in clinical practice, regardless of their clinical specialty. And they cover a broad spectrum of nursing activities, from disease prevention to health promotion and maintenance.

The ANA outlines a competent level of nursing care using six major standards. Each standard corresponds to a specific stage of the nursing process (in the ANA's model, the planning stage is divided into two discrete phases: outcome identifica-

Nursing standards and the courts

Even if they aren't law, nursing standards have important legal significance. The premise of any lawsuit against a nurse rests on suspected failure to meet appropriate standards of care.

During a legal dispute, the court will measure the defendant-nurse's action against the answer it obtains to the following question: What would a reasonably prudent nurse, with similar training and experience, do under similar conditions?

To answer this question, the plaintiff, through his attorney, must determine that certain standards of care exist and that the defendant-nurse should have applied those standards to him. He also must prove the appropriateness of those standards, show how the nurse failed to meet them, and show how this failure caused him injury.

Citing practice standards

The case of *Story v. St. Mary Parish Service District* (1987) shows how courts consider national standards of care. In this case, a 66-year-old man was admitted to the hospital complaining of abdominal distention and pain, nausea, and vomiting. Throughout the next 2 days, he complained several times to the nurses and attendants about shortness of breath and severe pain in his elbows and chest.

One evening, the staff nurse (a new graduate who had only recently taken her nursing board examination) wrote in her nurses' notes, "Complains of both elbows hurting severely, denied pain anywhere else. Slightly irritable and confused. Assisted back to bed. Admits to arthritis. Slight shortness of breath noted. Abdominal distention in moderation noted; soft to touch. Blood pressure 150/98; pulse 88. Will have (him) medicated." She did not indicate any consultation with the charge nurse. The patient died at 11:45 p.m.; the autopsy revealed a myocardial infarction.

Pretrial testimony revealed that the patient had stated that the nurses did not listen to his reports of pain. In the pretrial memorandum, the plaintiff's attorney cited various nursing practice standards, including the following:
• the Louisiana Nurse Practice Act, which describes the nurse's responsibility for assessing patients and intervening appropriately
• a board of nursing rule stating that graduate nurses must be supervised by a registered nurse when they provide care
• nursing care standards established by the JCAHO.

Although this case was settled out of court, it's a good example of the extensive use of nursing practice standards in a lawsuit.

National or local standards?

Although courts may consider national, state, and community standards when judging the quality of nursing care, national standards are gaining increased importance in negligence cases. That means both your expertise and performance must keep pace with national trends in nursing standards of care.

(continued)

Nursing standards and the courts – *continued*

In *Wickliffe v. Sunrise Hospital, Inc.* (1985), Angela Wickliffe's parents alleged that nursing negligence – violation of both written hospital procedures and accepted national standards of nursing care – caused their daughter's wrongful death.

After Angela Wickliffe, a healthy 13-year-old, underwent surgery to correct scoliosis of the spine, she received a narcotic antagonist to reverse the anesthesia. During her stay in the recovery room, she also was given 12 mg of morphine and 1 mg of diazepam (Valium) to minimize her restlessness.

At 11:20 a.m., when Angela was transferred from the recovery room to a surgical unit, the recovery room nurse reported the medications Angela had received to the head nurse. Because Angela's assigned nurse was at lunch, a patient care attendant checked her vital signs at 11:30 a.m. – they were normal. At 12:15 p.m., Angela's assigned nurse filled her water pitcher and noticed that she was snoring. At 12:30 p.m., when a nursing assistant took in a food tray, Angela was still snoring. The assistant left to check if Angela was to have lunch. On her return 10 minutes later, she discovered that Angela had no pulse or respirations.

Although Angela was revived to a comatose state, she died from brain damage 12 days later.

In their suit against the hospital, the Wickliffes pointed out that Angela's vital signs weren't checked between her return to the unit at 11:30 a.m. and the discovery of her respiratory arrest at 12:40 p.m. They argued that the hospital's policy and nursing standards of care require that a postoperative patient's vital signs be monitored every 15 minutes during the first hour after his return to the surgical unit.

A nurse expert witness testified for the Wickliffes that this lack of monitoring violated a national standard of nursing care and thus was negligence. She based her opinion on the level of care promulgated by the American College of Utilization Review Physicians and by the JCAHO as well as on her own familiarity with nursing procedures. The district court ruled that this nurse's testimony as an expert witness should be excluded because she was not familiar with practices in the locality in which the case occurred. The jury then returned a verdict in favor of the hospital.

This judgment was reversed on appeal. Noting that hospitals are accredited by the JCAHO, which establishes standards for all hospitals seeking accreditation, the court argued that national nursing standards do exist. The court also contended that nursing education and licensing are standardized: A nurse licensed in one state, for instance, can practice in another without taking the second state's licensing examination.

Thus, the court held that an expert witness who is familiar with the standard of care of a reasonably competent nurse in similar circumstances, regardless of location, may testify in a negligence action against a hospital or its employees. Determining whether circumstances are similar in a particular case is up to the jury.

At one time in negligence cases, a nurse's practice was evaluated against the standard of care of nurses practicing in the same geographic area. This "locality rule" reflected the wide disparity between the health care available in urban and rural settings. With advances in technology, communication, and transportation, however, this rule has become obsolete.

tion and planning). To meet the ANA standards, you'll need to provide a competent level of care for each stage of the nursing process.

Assessment
When you're collecting health data from a patient, the ANA expects you to set priorities for data collection according to the patient's immediate concerns and needs. You're required to collect pertinent data using the appropriate techniques and, when necessary, to involve the patient, family members, other caregivers, and health care providers. In addition, you must use a systematic and ongoing process to collect assessment data. Finally, you must document the relevant data in a retrievable form.

Nursing diagnosis
To meet ANA standards, you must derive your nursing diagnoses from analysis of the assessment data. You're expected to validate the diagnosis with your patient and, when possible, with family members, other caregivers, and health care providers. You should document your diagnosis in a way that facilitates identification of expected outcomes and formulation of the plan of care.

Outcome identification
To meet this standard, you must develop individualized expected outcomes for each patient. Derive your outcomes from the diagnoses, and document your outcomes as measurable goals. You should work with the patient and other health care providers to formulate outcomes. Also, make sure that the outcomes you develop reflect the patient's current and potential capabilities. Include a time frame for attaining outcomes, and provide direction for continuity of care.

Planning
Your plan of care should prescribe interventions to attain expected outcomes and should be tailored to your patient's needs and condition. It should also reflect current nursing practice. When developing the plan of care, work with the patient and, when appropriate, with family members, other caregivers, and health care providers. In addition, you must document your plan and provide for continuity of care.

Implementation

The ANA expects you to intervene safely and appropriately. To meet its standards, your interventions must be consistent with the established plan of care and must be documented.

Evaluation

Under ANA standards, you're required to evaluate the patient's progress in attaining outcomes. You should document the patient's responses to interventions and conduct systematic and ongoing evaluations. In addition, you're required to evaluate the effectiveness of interventions in relation to outcomes and use ongoing assessment data to revise nursing diagnoses, outcomes, and the plan of care, as needed. To meet this standard, you'll need to document revisions in nursing diagnoses, outcomes, and the plan of care. Finally, be sure to involve the patient, family members, other caregivers, and health care providers in the evaluation process, when appropriate.

National consensus

When developing practice standards, the ANA polls its national membership. Because the standards represent a national consensus, they carry considerable authority in court. Thus, in a legal dispute, your record of your actions may be compared to the expected level of practice, as defined by the national standards. If your documentation doesn't show that your actions met these standards, you increase your risk of liability.

JCAHO standards

A private, nonprofit organization, the JCAHO establishes standards and conducts voluntary accreditation programs for hospitals and other health care facilities. These facilities include psychiatric clinics and hospitals, substance abuse treatment and rehabilitation centers, community mental health centers, long-term care facilities, hospices, freestanding ambulatory care facilities, home care organizations, and centers for the developmentally disabled.

As part of its mission to improve the quality of public health care, the JCAHO has developed nursing care standards. Meeting these standards is important for two reasons. First, JCAHO standards provide general guidelines for meeting patient care needs and understanding current trends in health care delivery. Second, documenting according to JCAHO standards is necessary to ensure continued accreditation of your facility.

Unlike ANA standards, JCAHO standards aren't organized according to the nursing process. Instead, each standard states an expectation that must be met for accreditation. The JCAHO gives nurses considerable latitude in meeting its standards. More than one approach may work, as long as the standard's intent is fulfilled.

Documenting care accurately is key to meeting JCAHO standards. The standards require that you document evidence that the nursing process was used for each patient. However, the JCAHO standards don't dictate a format for documentation; that decision is left up to each hospital. (See *Choosing your charting format*, page 206.)

Other JCAHO standards pertain broadly to assessment, nursing diagnosis, and implementation.

Assessment
According to JCAHO standards, a registered nurse is responsible for assessing the nursing care needs of each patient admitted to the hospital. Although data collection may be performed by other qualified personnel — doctors, dietitians, licensed practical nurses, and physical therapists, for example — a registered nurse still must see the patient and validate the information. Assessment must be documented. When appropriate, the patient's family, friends, and other caregivers should be involved in the assessment process.

Under JCAHO guidelines, your hospital, if accredited, is obligated to establish a reasonable time for you to complete your admission assessment. You're also expected to reassess your patient periodically, depending on his condition and other factors. (See *JCAHO assessment timetables*, page 207.)

What to assess
During your assessment, the JCAHO expects you to consider a broad range of factors, including biophysical, psychosocial, environmental, self-care, educational, and discharge planning ones.

Assessing biophysical needs may include a review of major body systems (neurologic, cardiovascular, respiratory, and so on). Examples of physiologic assessment factors include vital signs, laboratory values, cardiac rhythm, neurologic status, respiratory capacity, and the presence of prostheses.

Choosing your charting format

Under JCAHO standards that went into effect in 1991, evidence that the nursing process has been used must be integrated into the patient's medical record. These standards require that the medical records of all patients who receive nursing care contain documentation of the following information:
• initial assessment by a registered nurse and subsequent reassessments
• nursing diagnoses or patient care needs or both
• plan of care or nursing standards of patient care used to address identified nursing diagnoses or patient care needs, including any interventions
• nursing care provided
• outcome of nursing interventions (the patient's response to interventions)
• ability of the patient (or his family) to manage continuing care needs after discharge.

Charting alternatives
JCAHO requirements state that all data related to patient assessments, the nursing care planned, nursing interventions, and patient outcomes must be "permanently integrated into the clinical information system."

Exactly what is a "clinical information system?" Broadly speaking, it's your hospital's method of recording and documenting patient care information. JCAHO standards do not require any specific medical record form or format. These new standards open the door to various charting alternatives, for example:
• critical paths—a day-by-day summary of the patient's stay in the hospital. Nurses and doctors collaborate to map the patient's daily need for consultations, activities, medications, diet, tests, and other elements of care.
• computerized plans of care—electronic patient charts that are replacing handwritten or typewritten plans at many hospitals. A patient's record may consist of handwritten and computer-generated forms.
• charting by exception—documentation of significant or abnormal findings; normal findings may be checked off on flow sheets and graphic records.
• PIE charting—use of the problem, implementation, and evaluation (PIE) format to document nursing notes.

Nursing information also can be presented in flow charts, tables, computer-generated graphics, or traditional narrative notes, among other formats.

Regardless of which format you work with, keep in mind these two JCAHO requirements: First, nursing information must be integrated into the medical record. Second, a reader of the record should be able to identify and retrieve nursing care data from the clinical information system, when necessary.

Examples of psychosocial factors include the patient's support systems, fears, anxiety, mental status, coping mecha-

JCAHO assessment timetables

JCAHO standards require that nursing care be based on a documented patient assessment. However, the timing of the assessment may vary according to the patient's needs. The JCAHO suggests the following time frames for completing an admission assessment. Specific guidelines can be found in your hospital policy manual.

TYPE OF PATIENT	TIMETABLE FOR COMPLETING ADMISSION ASSESSMENT
Critical care	5 to 10 minutes after admission
Labor	5 minutes after admission
Medical-surgical	8 hours after admission
Psychiatric	8 hours after admission
Rehabilitation	1 to 3 days before admission
Long-term care	3 days after admission
Pediatric	8 hours after admission
Emergency	On arrival

Reassessment guidelines
The JCAHO also suggests guidelines for reassessment. Keep in mind that a patient may need more frequent reassessment, depending on the urgency of his condition. Again, consult your hospital policy manual.

TYPE OF PATIENT	WHEN TO REASSESS
One with active GI bleeding	Continuously on a 1-to-1 basis
Suicidal	Continuously on a 1-to-1 basis
One with deteriorating neurologic status	Every 15 minutes
Labor	Every 15 minutes
Long-term care	Weekly
Rehabilitation	Every 2 weeks
Same-day surgery	On return from recovery room and immediately before discharge

nisms, spiritual values, sleep patterns, habits (such as alcohol and drug use), work history, and recreational activities.

When assessing environmental factors, you might ask the patient where he lives and whether he has access to continuing medical care. You might inquire about his socioeconomic status and general living conditions. Assess whether he requires special equipment, such as a walking cane.

Self-care and educational factors might include the patient's ability to carry out activities of daily living, the presence of physical or psychological impairment, and the need for home health assistance.

Be sure to assess the patient's discharge planning needs. You might also want to assess special learning needs and determine the need for modification to the home environment.

Nursing diagnosis

In 1991, the JCAHO took a major step by incorporating nursing diagnosis into its revised standards of care. The JCAHO now requires that a registered nurse base the patient's care on nursing diagnoses or another documented format, such as a problem list or a patient nursing care needs list. Other providers, such as licensed practical nurses and nursing assistants, can collect patient data, but only a registered nurse can formulate the nursing diagnoses or patient problem list.

Implementation

JCAHO standards stress the importance of keeping the patient and his family, friends, and other caregivers informed about and involved in nursing care. In addition, the standards call for you to collaborate with members of the health care team when making decisions about each patient's nursing care needs. The patient's medical record should reflect this interdisciplinary approach, when appropriate, and nursing care should be consistent with therapies provided by other members of the health care team. Examples of interdisciplinary collaboration include team conferences and integrated charting.

JCAHO standards recognize the nurse's key role in patient education. You're expected to provide teaching that's specific to the patient's needs and that involves the patient's family, friends, and other caregivers, when appropriate. The medical record should show that the patient's learning needs have been identified and that nursing interventions have taken these needs into account. When addressing the patient's learning needs, you should consider the patient's anticipated length of stay, the nature and complexity of the patient's and family's learning needs, appropriate use of resources, and the patient's and family's ability to comprehend and implement teaching.

The patient's postdischarge needs must be assessed before he leaves the hospital. Document any referrals for postdischarge care in the patient's medical record.

LEGAL ASPECTS OF DOCUMENTATION

Documentation provides legal proof of the nature and quality of care that the patient received. The weight that the medical record—the principal tool used by the health care team to plan, coordinate, and document care—carries in legal proceedings can't be overemphasized. The patient's medical record may be the focus of inquiry in personal injury, professional malpractice, or product liability claims. For example, under the diagnosis-related group (DRG) system, patients are at risk for being discharged prematurely and injured as a result; therefore, thorough documentation of a patient's readiness for discharge is crucial. The medical record may be used as evidence in other types of cases, such as workers' compensation, child custody, and employment disputes.

All health care professionals have a legal duty to maintain the medical record in sufficient detail because inadequate documentation of care could result in liability or nonreimbursement by third-party payers. In effect, the general rule that "what isn't in the record didn't occur" continues to dominate.

As part of the permanent medical record, nursing documentation must be factual, consistent, timely, and complete. Usually, your facility's policy and procedure manual will describe how and what to document. To legally protect yourself and your institution, you should document the following information:

• initial assessment data and applicable nursing diagnoses
• nursing actions, including interventions and reports to the doctor
• ongoing assessment, including the frequency of reassessment
• variations from the assessment and plan of care
• accountability information, including forms signed by the patient and the location of his valuables
• notation of care by other health care professionals, including the doctor's visits, if practical
• patient teaching, including content and response
• procedures and diagnostic tests
• patient response to therapy, particularly to nursing interventions, and diagnostic tests
• statements made by the patient
• patient comfort and safety measures
• discharge planning guidelines, if relevant.

Hazards of improper documentation

In the past, nurses and other health care providers made documentation errors that contributed substantially to the verdict in lawsuits. To avoid making the same mistakes, review the following court cases about faulty record keeping, failure to include information, charting after the fact, and missing records. All of these cases contain important lessons about the courts' determination to uphold standards of documentation.

Faulty records

Rogers v. Kasdan (1981) involved a woman who died of brain damage 7 days after her admission to the hospital for injuries sustained in an accident. In the lawsuit that followed, the Supreme Court of Kentucky ruled against the doctor and the hospital. The court based its ruling on the patient's medical record: The emergency department records were incomplete, the fluid intake and output record was incorrectly tallied, various records contained discrepancies, and several records were illegible and contained incomplete notations.

Absence of information

St. Paul Fire and Marine Insurance Co. v. Prothro (1979) involved a claim in which the patient, after undergoing a total hip replacement, was injured while being lowered into a Hubbard tank by an orderly. The metal basket holding him collapsed, his hip was struck, and his wound reopened. The orderly stopped the bleeding and took the plaintiff to his room, where a nurse treated the wound. However, the nurse failed to document the incident. The wound subsequently became infected, necessitating the removal of the prosthesis and leaving the patient with a permanent limp. The court ruled in the patient's favor and noted that a determining factor was the absence in the patient's medical chart of critical information that would have assisted the doctor and staff in providing proper care.

Charting after the fact

In *Joseph Brant Memorial Hospital v. Koziol* (1978), a nurse failed to chart her observations for 7 hours on a postoperative patient who died during that period. The patient's family sued the hospital, claiming nursing malpractice. The nurse insisted that she had observed the patient and, on the instruction of the assistant director of nursing, had added nursing observations to the patient's medical record after the fact. Citing the altered record, the court ruled that the nurse's failure to chart her observations at the proper time supported the claim that she had made no such observations.

In another case, *Thor v. Boska* (1974), a rewritten copy of a patient's record was suspected of being an altered record. This lawsuit involved a woman who had seen her doctor several times because of a breast lump. Each time, the doctor examined her and made a record of her visit. After 2 years, the woman sought a second opinion and learned that she had breast cancer. She sued her first doctor. But rather than producing his records in court, the doctor brought copies of the records and said he had copied the originals for legibility. The court reasoned that he was withholding incriminating evidence and found in favor of the plaintiff.

Missing records

The case of *Battocchi v. Washington Hospital Center* (1990) underscores the significance of missing records. In this case, parents brought a malpractice suit against the hospital and a doctor for injuries that their son sustained during forceps delivery. The nurse in attendance documented the events and her observations of the delivery immediately after the delivery, and posted the record in the chart.

Later the hospital's risk management personnel obtained the chart for analysis and, apparently, lost the nurse's record. The court entered judgment in favor of the hospital and doctor, holding that the jury couldn't presume negligence and causation against them simply because the hospital lost the nurses' notes. But the District of Columbia Court of Appeals sent the case back to the trial court so that it could rule whether the hospital's loss of the records stemmed from negligence or impropriety.

Avoiding documentation errors

Besides their potential impact on patient care, charting errors or omissions, even if seemingly harmless, will undermine your credibility in court. Especially watch out for omissions, inclusion of personal opinions, vague or late entries, and various other problems described in the following paragraphs.

Omissions

Include all facts that other nurses will need to assess the patient. In a lawsuit, the court may conclude that a nurse failed to perform a nursing action that's absent from the record or that data were omitted with the intent of obscuring incriminating evidence.

Personal opinions
Don't enter personal opinions or speculative remarks as to what presumably occurred. Record only factual and objective observations and findings as well as the patient's actual statements.

Vague entries
Don't generalize or record vague or ambiguous observations. Be specific, avoiding such entries as "Patient had a good day." Instead, describe why the patient's day was good: "Patient ate 100% of regular diet; did not complain of pain."

Late entries
Record patient data in a timely manner. But if a late entry is necessary, identify it as such and sign and date the entry in accordance with your facility's policy.

Improper corrections
Never erase or obliterate an error. Draw a single line through the error so that it remains legible, label it "error," and sign and date the correction.

Erroneous or unclear abbreviations
Use only standard and accepted abbreviations in common usage, and follow your facility's policies and procedures. Whenever you're in doubt, spell out the abbreviation. Common abbreviations, even if standardized, should be documented in your facility's policy and procedure manual. All staff members, both permanent and temporary, should be aware of which abbreviations are acceptable.

Illegibility and lack of clarity
Be sure to write so that others can read your entry. Use common terms and expressions, and consult a dictionary if you're unsure of a term's spelling or usage.

Unsigned entries
Sign all notes with your first initial, full last name, and title. Place your signature on the right side of the page as proof that you entered all the information between the previous nurse's signature and your own. If the last entry is unsigned, contact

the nurse who made the entry and request the signature. Draw lines through empty or remaining spaces to prevent subsequent amendments or additions.

Be sure to countersign only those entries that you can validate with the member of the health care team who provided the "hands-on care." Make sure you're familiar with your facility's policies and procedures for countersigning.

Suspicious changes

In the event of a legal challenge, you should never retrospectively change, correct, or add to the documented record. To do so would raise suspicion, even if you have a legitimate reason for making the change and the best of intentions. If you need to keep records when you know that a legal question is pending, keep a private log concerning the patient's care.

KEY POINTS

• Nursing care standards set minimum criteria for nursing proficiency. Becoming aware of these standards will help you judge the quality of care you and your nursing colleagues provide.
• Nursing standards have important legal significance, even if they aren't law. The premise of every nursing negligence or malpractice lawsuit is that a nurse failed to meet minimum standards of care. The courts are increasingly relying on national standards of care in deciding legal disputes.
• As the professional association for registered nurses, the ANA is responsible for developing standards of care for all practicing nurses. ANA standards are generic–they apply to all registered nurses in clinical practice, regardless of their clinical specialty.
• In its revised *Standards of Clinical Nursing Practice,* the ANA describes a competent level of nursing care using six major standards. Each standard corresponds to a specific stage of the nursing process.
• The JCAHO has developed nursing standards that are used when auditing a health care facility during an accreditation survey. The standards require you to document evidence that the nursing process was used for each patient. However, the JCAHO standards don't dictate a format for documentation; that decision is left to each hospital.

• New JCAHO standards allow use of newer documentation formats, such as charting by exception, critical paths, PIE charting, and computerized charting.

• In 1991, the JCAHO incorporated nursing diagnosis into its revised standards of care. The JCAHO now requires that a registered nurse base the patient's care on nursing diagnoses or another documented format, such as a problem list or a patient nursing care needs list.

• The medical record provides legal proof of the nature and quality of care that the patient received. The weight it carries in legal proceedings is enormous. Inadequate documentation of care may result in liability or nonreimbursement by third-party payers. The general rule that "what isn't in the record didn't occur" continues to dominate.

• If you ever become involved in a legal challenge, documentation errors could destroy your credibility in court. Follow these rules: Be careful to avoid omissions, don't enter personal opinions, avoid making vague or late entries, make corrections properly, use only standard and accepted abbreviations, write legibly, sign all entries, and avoid suspicious changes.

SELF-TEST

1. Which of the following statements about nursing standards is false?

   a. The American Nurses' Association (ANA) established the first generic standards for the profession in 1973.

   b. Courts are increasingly using professional standards to decide legal disputes involving nurses.

   c. Once established and accepted by the nursing profession, standards are rarely changed.

   d. Hospitals use nursing standards to measure patient outcomes and evaluate quality of care.

2. Under the standards of the Joint Commission on Accreditation of Healthcare Organizations (JCAHO), which of the following formats may you use to document your nursing care?

   a. problem-intervention-evaluation (PIE) format

   b. charting by exception

   c. narrative charting

   d. all of the above

3. According to JCAHO recommendations, how often should you reassess a patient receiving long-term care?

a. every 8 hours

b. every 24 hours

c. weekly

d. JCAHO guidelines don't provide a schedule for reassessing a patient receiving long-term care.

4. If you're ever a defendant in a malpractice or negligence suit, your actions will be compared with:

a. the actions of any qualified health care professional in a similar situation.

b. the actions of a reasonably prudent nurse in a similar situation.

c. the actions of a nurse with a similar or more advanced education.

d. the reasonable expectations of the patient, as stated under oath.

5. What do JCAHO standards have to say about nursing diagnoses?

a. They do not mention nursing diagnoses; this indicates that diagnosis will no longer be part of nursing practice by the end of the decade.

b. They state that a registered nurse should formulate a nursing diagnosis or a patient problem list for each patient but that this information should not be integrated into the medical record.

c. They require that each patient must be assigned at least one nursing diagnosis and that only terminology approved by the North American Nursing Diagnosis Association may be included in the medical record.

d. They require that each patient's care be based on identified nursing diagnoses or another documented format, such as a patient problem list.

6. If you make a mistake in a clinical record, you should:

a. white it out, then sign and date it.

b. leave it alone to avoid suspicion of tampering with records.

c. draw a single line through it, write "error" above or beside it, and sign and date your corrections.

d. erase it completely, write in the correct information, and initial and date the entry.

7. According to ANA standards, which of the following is *not* a requirement for patient outcome identification?
   a. Outcomes must be realistic in relation to the patient's capabilities.
   b. Outcomes are derived from assessment data.
   c. Outcomes are revised according to ongoing assessment findings.
   d. Outcomes should include a time estimate for attainment.

8. ANA standards carry significant weight in legal disputes because they:
   a. have the binding power of statutory law.
   b. affect both licensed practical nurses and registered nurses.
   c. represent a national consensus.
   d. were the first set of standards to be accepted by the majority of nurses.

9. Mary Novacek, RN, works the 3-to-11 p.m. shift and forgot to document that she took Mr. Green's vital signs at 4 p.m. It's now the end of her shift and she realizes her mistake. Which of the following actions is most appropriate?
   a. Ms. Novacek should document the missing information neatly and sign it.
   b. She should document the missing information and identify it as a late entry.
   c. She should inform her supervisor of her mistake and document an incident report.
   d. She should record the mistake in her personal log.

10. In cases of nursing negligence, which of the following is generally true?
    a. National standards are being favored over local and state standards.
    b. The locality rule continues to dominate.
    c. Nurses do not have "deep pockets" and therefore are rarely named in lawsuits.

d. Nurses who provide appropriate care and document accurately won't be sued.

(For answers with rationales, turn to page 264.)

FURTHER READINGS

Accreditation Manual for Hospitals, 2 vols. Oakbrook Terrace, Ill.: Joint Commission on Accreditation of Healthcare Organizations, 1993.

An Introduction to Joint Commission Nursing Care Standards. Oakbrook Terrace, Ill.: Joint Commission on Accreditation of Healthcare Organizations, 1991.

Clark, M.D. "Toward Safer Nursing Practice," *Nursing Management* 22(3):88-90, March 1991.

Fiesta, J. "Look Beyond Your State for Your Standards of Care," *Nursing86* 16(8):66, August 1986.

Fiesta, J. "QA and Risk Management: Reducing Liability Exposure," *Nursing Management* 22(2):14-15, February 1991.

Fiesta, J. "Safeguarding Your Nursing License," *Nursing Management* 21(8):20-21, August 1990.

Killian, W.H. "Nurses Face Increasing Liability," *American Nurse* 22(1):43, January 1990.

Kraus, N. "Malpractice Litigation: A Painful Lesson in Professional Responsibility," *Journal of Nurse-Midwifery* 35(3):125-26, May-June 1990.

Lacombe, D.C. "Avoiding a Malpractice Nightmare," *Nursing90* 20(6):42-43, June 1990.

Luquire, R. "Nursing Risk Management," *Nursing Management* 20(10):56-58, October 1989.

McMullen, P. "On the Nature of a Malpractice Suit—A Thumbnail Overview," *Nursing Connections* 2(4):51-52, Winter 1989.

Murphy, E.K. "Legal Concerns of the Next Decade," *AORN Journal* 51(1):258-61, January 1990.

Nurse's Handbook of Law and Ethics. Springhouse, Pa.: Springhouse Corp., 1992.

Standards of Clinical Nursing Practice. Kansas City, Mo.: American Nurses' Association, 1991.

CHAPTER 9

COMPUTERS AND THE NURSING PROCESS

Someday soon, the traditional handwritten patient chart may become a relic of nursing history. Its successor: a computer-generated electronic chart that allows nurses to collect, display, and store patient information with a few swift touches to a keyboard. Paperless charting represents just one of the benefits computers offer to nurses, however. Increasingly, nurses are using computers to increase efficiency and accuracy in every phase of the nursing process.

Computers, of course, are nothing new in the health care industry. For years, hospitals have used them for payrolls, billing, patient bed assignments, pharmacy orders, and auxiliary needs. What's more, many facilities use specially designed software programs called "hospital information systems" to link various departments electronically. But nursing departments typically have been among the last to use computers to meet their needs.

Why? Largely because the software programs that can handle the complex requirements of nursing departments have not been available until recently. Also, nurses haven't traditionally participated in organizational decisions about the implementation of technology. Nor have nurses always agreed on the type of nursing data to include in hospital information systems. In addition, because computers are expensive, administrators have been reluctant to invest in them until they were sure that the technology would save nurses time and hospitals money.

But as you'll discover in this chapter, nurses are catching up fast. A growing number of progressive health care facilities have installed computerized nursing information systems (NISs) to collect, process, and communicate data used by nurses in the delivery of patient care. If you aren't using a computer yet, chances are you will be soon.

This chapter will help you become familiar with computers and show you how these devices can assist with each phase of the nursing process. You'll also learn how to adapt to a new computer system and explore the advantages and disadvantages of automated technology. And you'll review some of the exciting new developments in computer use and technology — developments bound to have a tremendous effect on the future of nursing.

BECOMING FAMILIAR WITH COMPUTERS

Before using a computer, you'll need to become familiar with its functions and learn some commonly used computer terms. (See *Understanding computer terms*, page 220.) To use a hospital information system, you enter a code or the patient's name to bring the patient's chart onto the screen. You then select the function you want. For example, you can enter new data on the nursing plan of care or progress notes, or review vital signs for comparison. You can perform these activities more quickly than you could using handwritten or typed documentation.

Depending on the computer's type and software, you may enter information using a keyboard, a light pen, a touch-sensitive screen, a mouse, or even your voice. One emerging technology, pen-based input, allows your writing to be stored as data. Your facility may use various computers. For example, a large mainframe computer can provide centralized data storage for all departments. Personal computers or terminals located at work stations throughout the facility can allow access to this information. Also, many hospitals now provide terminals right at patients' bedsides. (See *Bedside computers*, page 221.)

If your facility uses an NIS, you can record nursing actions directly into the electronic record. This system supports most or all nursing process steps. It can help you to meet the nursing care standards established by the American Nurses' Association (ANA) and the Joint Commission on Accreditation of Healthcare Organizations (JCAHO). What's more, each NIS can be customized to meet the specific needs of your facility or nursing department.

Most NISs manage information passively; that is, they can collect, display, and store data, but they usually can't recommend or make clinical decisions. The more sophisticated systems provide you with a selection of standardized phrases for documenting patient status and nursing interventions. You

Understanding computer terms

To understand hospital computer systems better, you'll need to become familiar with basic computer terminology. Here are some common computer terms and their definitions.

Central processing unit (CPU) • Part of a computer where arithmetic and logical functions are performed and instructions are decoded and executed. The CPU directs the computer's operation.

Computer • Electronic machine that operates under the control of instructions stored in its memory unit. These instructions allow the machine to accept and store data and perform other logical operations.

Computer hardware • Basic operating parts of the computer, such as the disk drives and the microprocessor.

Computer program • Also called computer software, a series of instructions that tell a computer how to perform various tasks, such as retrieving information, performing calculations, and conducting data searches.

Data base • Collection of data (factual information) organized so as to facilitate retrieval and use.

Data security and control • Safeguards in the computer system that allow only authorized personnel to read or otherwise use stored data.

Diskette • Also called a floppy disk, a plastic disk, commonly used in personal computers, that stores data as magnetic spots.

Download • To transmit a file or program from a large computer to a smaller one.

Electronic data processing • Also called information processing, the production of information by processing data on a computer.

Mainframe • Large, centralized computer that can store vast volumes of data and provide access to numerous users.

Microcomputer • Also called a personal computer or a PC, a small computer with less memory capacity and slower processing speeds than the larger mainframe.

Microprocessor • Integrated circuit containing the entire CPU of a computer.

Network • Information system formed by electronically linking two or more computers or terminals.

On-line system • System in which data are entered into a device, such as a terminal, that is connected directly to a computer.

Password • Secret code that allows a user to gain access to the computer.

Response time • Duration between the moment a user enters data and the moment the computer responds to the entry.

Time-sharing • Method of running more than one program on a single computer that allows many users at different terminals to be served simultaneously.

User friendly • Easy to learn and use; often said of software that can be used by people with limited training or experience.

can revise these standardized phrases or insert your own narrative notes to individualize information.

Bedside computers

Bedside terminals bring computer power and efficiency directly to each patient's room. Also known as point-of-care (POC) systems, bedside computer terminals have been installed in hospitals and other clinical settings, such as nursing homes. With a bedside terminal, you can document assessment data as soon as you acquire it and record patient care as you provide it. No longer do you need to write on a work sheet and later copy the information onto the patient's chart.

A bedside computer typically consists of a standard video monitor and a keyboard. Usually, terminals are connected to the main computer at the nurses' station, which in turn is linked to a network of other computers throughout the hospital. The exact configuration of POC systems varies from one health care facility to the next. In some settings, the terminals are equipped with simplified keyboards that have about 20 keys, each of which is labeled with some aspect of the patient care process, such as patient teaching. With these systems, you need only press a button to view any portion of a patient's chart. However, you may need to use another terminal with a standard keyboard to enter additional narrative notes.

A time-saver
Studies show that nurses spend up to half of their time in documentation; bedside systems streamline the process by making data entry more efficient. At some hospitals, charting time has been reduced by at least one half hour per nurse per shift. Bedside computers also are convenient. Unlike the computer at the nursing station, which may be occupied constantly, the bedside computer usually is available when needed.

A bedside computer can free you to spend more time with your patients. While charting, for example, you can talk to the patient and family and answer their questions. The terminal also helps to improve patient care by reminding you to collect and document appropriate assessment data.

Patients often appreciate bedside computers as well. Because all aspects of the medical record are stored in the electronic data base, the patient is spared the repetitious questioning from a series of health care providers, all seeking the same information. Also, hospital staff members in different departments can simultaneously view the same patient's chart, provided that enough terminals exist.

A well-designed system can promote nursing recruitment and retention. In fact, after working with POC systems, some nurses say they wouldn't want to work anywhere that didn't offer electronic charting.

Potential drawbacks
You'll need to reassure patients that the system contains safeguards to prevent electronic invasion of their privacy. And from a technical perspective, some systems run too slowly because they lack adequate "memory" or data storage space. This inefficiency, if not corrected, may cause nurses to return to traditional charting.

USING COMPUTERS IN THE NURSING PROCESS

An NIS can be either a stand-alone system or a subsystem of a larger hospital information system. In either case, this technology can help you implement each nursing process step.

Assessment

In a typical scenario, you begin assessing your patient by turning on the computer terminal to record admission information. As you collect information on the patient's health status, history, chief complaint, and other assessment factors, you type it into the computer.

Some software programs prompt you to ask specific assessment questions and, depending on your answers, lead you down various pathways, or "decision trees," to gather further information. In some systems, if you enter an assessment value that's beyond the usual acceptable range, the computer will flag the entry to call your attention to it.

Nursing diagnosis

After you've collected the pertinent assessment data, you're ready to formulate appropriate nursing diagnoses. Computer programs that propose diagnoses are still experimental. Currently, most programs list standard diagnoses along with associated assessment findings. You still must rely on your clinical judgment to determine the appropriate nursing diagnoses for each patient.

However, a computer can provide you with more rapid access to nursing diagnosis information. For example, you can use a computer to quickly generate a list of possible nursing diagnoses for a patient with selected assessment findings. You can also use a computer to store and sort patient records by nursing diagnosis. This would allow you to enter a nursing diagnosis and have the computer print out records of all patients with that nursing diagnosis. Thus, using a computer can improve accuracy in selecting nursing diagnoses. In addition, because the list of nursing diagnoses can change every 2 years, a computer can help you stay current.

Planning

By displaying recommended expected outcomes and interventions for selected nursing diagnoses, computers can ease the difficulty and frustration nurses experience when they encounter blank care-planning formats. The computer can also be used to revise the plan of care.

In the future, computers may play a greater role in planning patient care. Because computers can track outcomes for large patient populations, computer-based research may be used to compare large amounts of patient data, thereby facilitating the selection of appropriate expected outcomes. With the development of large nursing data bases and sophisticated decision support software, computers eventually may help you determine which outcomes the patient is likely to attain — and when.

Implementation
Automated patient monitoring, especially in such areas as the coronary care and intensive care units, can greatly enhance your ability to perform timely nursing interventions. Computer-generated progress notes — which automatically sort and print out patient data (such as medication administration times, treatments, and vital signs) daily — can make documentation of the implementation phase more efficient and accurate. You can also use the computer to record your interventions as well as patient-processing information, such as transfer and discharge instructions, and to communicate this information to other hospital departments.

Evaluation
Although this phase of the nursing process requires your critical analysis to judge the patient's response to nursing interventions, you can use the computer to write and store your observations, the patient's response to nursing interventions, and your evaluation statements.

In the future, computer-based research may be used to facilitate retrospective evaluation of care. Using computer technology, you can compare patient records to determine which interventions provide optimal outcomes for patients with a particular nursing diagnosis. Over time, analysis of this information may help determine the most effective interventions and weed out less effective ones. Researchers are currently developing patient outcomes to include in nursing data bases that will be used to facilitate evaluation of quality of care.

ADAPTING TO A NEW COMPUTER SYSTEM
Computerization entails new ways of handling information, which can create changes in nursing roles, responsibilities, and relationships. Some nurses may feel like "computer illiterates" and either refuse to learn the new technology or de-

Questions to ask computer vendors

If your hospital is planning to install a nursing information system, here are some questions that should be addressed to computer vendors:
• Does the nursing information system have the capacity to store large amounts of clinical data?
• Does the system encode data so that it can be used in statistical analysis?
• Can the system retrieve data in sufficient clinical detail? Alternatively, can the system be modified to limit the amount of data generated to enable the user to focus on essential information?
• Will the system generate patient data in chronological order?
• Will electronic flow sheets represent how doctors and nurses actually deliver care?
• Will the system generate formatted and guided displays that enable the nurse to conveniently enter patient assessment data and develop a plan of care, progress notes, and discharge summaries?
• Will formatted documentation programs allow the nurse to enter personal notes to individualize care?
• Will the system's clinical data coding ensure simple, quick retrieval?
• Can the system communicate directly with computer systems of other departments, such as the laboratory, pharmacy, and radiology department, so that current information is always available?

clare themselves unable to learn it. Others may fear that they'll be replaced by a computer. Such fears may interfere with the successful integration of computers into a nursing department.

Education is the key to allaying fears about computers. The benefits of installing an NIS should be clearly explained to all staff members. Describing successful experiences that nurses in other hospitals have had with computer systems may help overcome resistance.

If your department is planning to install an NIS, you may want to ask your staff development office to arrange one or more seminars to orient the nursing staff to computer hardware and terminology. Also, some hospitals maintain personal-computing learning centers, where nurses and other staff members can acquire direct, hands-on experience. Alternatively, you may want to set up a regular forum, such as a monthly lunchtime seminar, where nurses can meet to air questions, concerns, and comments about using a new computer system. Nursing staff, through its leadership, should play a significant role in determining what type of NIS software and hardware your facility installs. (See *Questions to ask computer vendors.*)

Perhaps most important, if you're not an experienced computer user, give yourself time to learn. Although you may learn a computer's basic functions quickly, you'll need time to feel truly comfortable with computer charting and other sophisticated applications. If you feel uncertain about your computer skills, try double-charting on one patient for a few days; then see how your electronic chart compares to your traditional handwritten chart.

Advantages of computerization

The more nurses recognize what computers can do for them, the more likely they are to accept and apply computer technology in their practice. Because computers store and retrieve large amounts of information quickly and easily, they can make the nursing process more efficient, thereby freeing nurses to spend more time meeting the needs of their patients.

If your computer system is electronically linked with other departments, you can send or receive updated patient information instantly. For example, the computer can automatically notify the dietary department of diet changes, the pharmacy of new or revised medication orders, and the radiology department of X-ray requests. By disseminating information quickly, the computer helps to promote communication among nurses, doctors, and other staff members. This communication helps to ensure that your patient receives well-coordinated care.

Computers also decrease documentation errors, thereby reducing your risk of malpractice or negligence liability. By improving legibility, computers lessen the risk that your charting data will be misinterpreted. And because computers use standard terms and phrases, they promote better communication and allow more accurate comparison of data.

In addition, information stored in a computer is a valuable source of data on patient populations. Because computers use standardized formats, they allow you to make comparisons within and across various patient populations. You can use this information when conducting research or performing quality assurance studies.

A well-designed computer system connects patient assessment data with nursing diagnoses and the plan of care. This increases the likelihood that all nursing process steps will be fully implemented and documented, which enhances communication among nurses.

Disadvantages of computerization

Critics fear that computers will diminish the personal satisfaction that nurses derive from their practice. Technical advances, they argue, tend to have a dehumanizing effect on the work place. Relying on the computer may mean less opportunity for interaction and communication with co-workers and patients. If your patient believes that the computer, rather than his health care team, controls his care, he may become angry, cynical, fearful, or dependent and passive. Likewise, some nurses may substitute the reward they get from mastering computer technology for the satisfaction of patient care.

The computer's ability to retrieve data rapidly may prove too much of a good thing. If your computer inundates you with too much data, you may miss important information. In many cases, this problem can be resolved by modifying the software program or refining data-searching skills.

In addition, computerized assessment may threaten a patient's right to privacy if appropriate measures aren't taken to protect data. Your patient may be reluctant to divulge personal information if he feels that his history could be read by others without his knowledge or permission.

To protect your patient's right to privacy and ensure the confidentiality of his records, your computer system needs to have some safeguards. The primary safeguard is the signature code. By developing a series of access codes, programmers can limit access to the records. For example, a nurse's code might permit access to a patient's entire record, but a dietitian's code might produce only diet orders and the patient's nutrition history. If your patient expresses concern about an electronic breech of his privacy, explain the safeguards used at your facility.

Just like any other electronic device, computers occasionally break down, making information unavailable for indeterminate periods. Computers can also scramble patient information at times because of machine failure or human error. For this reason, your facility should have a backup system.

NEW DEVELOPMENTS

Important new developments include the emergence of nursing informatics as a distinct specialty and the development of the Nursing Minimum Data Set. In addition, technological advances, such as interactive programs, computerized medical libraries, and artificial intelligence, may profoundly affect nursing practice.

Nursing informatics

Nursing informatics integrates nursing and computer science with the goal of identifying, collecting, processing, and managing data to support nursing practice. In recent years, nursing informatics has emerged as an important discipline in its own right. For example, in January 1992 the ANA's Congress on Nursing Practice approved the designation of nursing informatics as a nursing specialty. The National League for Nursing has a Council for Nursing Informatics, which has begun preliminary work on developing educational curricula in this area.

Nursing Minimum Data Set

Leaders in the field of nursing informatics are seeking to have a greater role in determining what type of information is included in national health care data bases. These nurses believe that gaining access to nationwide nursing data is crucial to guiding the destiny of the profession.

For example, considerable work has already been done in the development and implementation of the Nursing Minimum Data Set (NMDS) — a system for standardizing the collection of essential nursing data. NMDS elements include the types of information used by the majority of nurses in all kinds of health care settings, such as nursing diagnoses, patient outcomes, nursing interventions, and patient demographics. Once collected, this information is stored in retrievable form on a computer data base.

If the NMDS were adopted nationwide (or worldwide), it would have far-reaching implications for nursing practice. It would enhance the consistency of nursing documentation by establishing national (or universal) standards for data collection and would facilitate comparison of nursing data from different clinical settings, patient populations, and geographic areas. By providing comparable nursing data on a large scale, the NMDS would lead to a more precise understanding of what nurses do, what they contribute to health care, and at what cost. NMDS data could also be used to demonstrate or project trends in nursing care and the allocation of nursing resources.

Large-scale implementation of the NMDS would help nurses gain greater influence in making health policy decisions. After all, tremendous amounts of information pertaining to clinical practice are contained in nursing documentation. Obtaining access to aggregate data derived from this documentation would be a powerful tool for influencing policy.

By developing links to information stored in NISs, the NMDS would stimulate nursing research. For example, NMDS data could be used to validate the defining characteristics of nursing diagnoses, thereby leading to more accurate diagnosis. The North American Nursing Diagnosis Association includes numerical codes with all of its nursing diagnoses so that diagnostic information can be entered into a computer.

The idea for a basic set of nursing data elements was conceived by Dr. Harriet Werley and colleagues at the 1979 University of Illinois Nursing Information System Conference. In 1985, a Nursing Minimum Data Set Conference was held at the University of Wisconsin at Milwaukee. In 1991, the ANA endorsed the NMDS as the essential nursing data elements that should be included in health care data bases and patient records. Although a number of health care facilities now include NMDS data in their information systems, more research by nurses into the implementation of the NMDS is needed. NMDS proponents hope that in the long run, the NMDS will become part of the information required by the federal government from health care providers who apply for Medicare reimbursement. This would help to ensure NMDS data collection on a broad scale.

Interactive programs

Information technology to support nursing practice continues to advance. The latest generation of NISs interacts with you, prompting you with questions and suggestions while you enter information about a patient. Sequential questioning and diagnostic suggestions generated by the computer make documentation thorough and quick, and provide assistance with decision making. Such programs allow you to add or change information as needed.

Although interactive programs are already being used in some areas, more work needs to be done to expedite development and implementation of this technology. Input from nurses into this process is crucial to ensure that interactive programs are efficient and accurate.

Computerized medical libraries

Advances in information technology will allow nurses to tap directly into computerized medical libraries. As you plan a patient's care or evaluate his responses to therapy, you'll be able to look up relevant journal articles or book passages through on-line library systems. Although limited, this capability is already available in some clinical settings.

Artificial intelligence

The advent of artificial intelligence may also enhance nursing practice. Still in the formative stage, artificial intelligence is a branch of computer science in which computers are used to simulate human thinking. The goal of those developing artificial intelligence is to create computer programs that can solve problems creatively rather than simply working through the steps of a solution designed by the programmer. For example, using expert systems technology, a computer program could be developed to emulate the thinking process of an experienced nurse practitioner in formulating nursing diagnoses and arriving at patient outcomes and nursing interventions. Other nurses would then be able to input patient data into this program and get expert advice on planning care.

Currently, researchers are investigating how to capture the knowledge of nursing experts and how to represent that knowledge in computer software programs. This task is complicated by the fact that much of nursing practice is focused on the qualitative aspects of health care—for example, performing psychosocial interventions and providing holistic care—and is difficult to translate into the quantitive language understood by computers. Another difficulty is reconciling the different views of various experts on clinical topics.

Developing expert systems is one of many challenges in adapting computer technology to meet the needs of contemporary nursing practice. Increasingly, computers will be used to help nurses make clinical decisions that are based on empirical evidence and creative and systematic thinking rather than on trial and error.

• Computerized nursing information systems support most or all nursing process steps. They can help you to meet the nursing care standards established by the ANA and the JCAHO.

• Bedside computer terminals allow nurses to document assessment information and nursing actions promptly.

• When computers are first used on a hospital unit, some nurses may refuse to learn the new technology or declare themselves unable to learn it. Others may fear that they'll be replaced by a computer. Such fears may interfere with the successful integration of computers into a nursing department. Education is the key to allaying these fears.

• Advantages of using computers in nursing include fast storage and retrieval of patient information; quicker, more efficient documentation; increased legibility of patient records; and enhanced ability to store large amounts of information on patient populations.

• Disadvantages of using computers include patients' fears of breached confidentiality, nurse-users becoming overwhelmed by excessive amounts of computer-generated data and, possibly, dehumanizing effects on the work place.

• The NMDS is a system for standardizing the collection of essential nursing data and storing these data in retrievable form on a computer data base. Nationwide implementation of the NMDS could make information on patient demographics, patient outcomes, use of nursing diagnoses, and other nursing data available on an unprecedented scale. It would facilitate comparison of nursing data from different clinical settings, patient populations, and geographic areas.

SELF-TEST

1. Using a nursing information system (NIS) can assist which of the following nursing activities?

    a. collecting assessment data
    b. developing a plan of care
    c. documenting progress notes
    d. all of the above

2. To gain entry to a patient's computerized clinical record, a nurse must enter a personal password or identifying data known as a:

a. signature code.
b. data entry sequence.
c. retrieval sequence.
d. user access sequence.

3. Which of the following statements best describes the computer's relationship to nursing diagnoses?

a. Current software packages do not include nursing diagnoses — an indication that diagnoses may eventually fade from clinical practice.
b. Current programs can analyze assessment data to determine appropriate nursing diagnoses.
c. Current programs can provide lists of diagnoses along with associated assessment findings.
d. Current software packages have a limited ability to select appropriate physiologic nursing diagnoses (such as decreased cardiac output) but cannot select appropriate behavioral diagnoses (such as ineffective individual coping).

4. Computer terminals installed at the patient's bedside are also know as:

a. information networks.
b. point-of-care systems.
c. hospital information systems.
d. nursing care networks.

5. Which of the following terms describes a collection of data in a form that facilitates retrieval and use of information?

a. artificial intelligence
b. downloading
c. data base
d. network

6. Which of the following terms describes an integrated circuit containing the entire central processing unit of a computer?

a. microprocessor
b. disk drive

c. byte
d. network

7. Of the computer types listed below, which can provide access to numerous users simultaneously?
   a. mainframe
   b. minicomputer
   c. microcomputer
   d. point-of-care terminal

8. All of the following statements describe the benefits of computers *except:*
   a. Computers improve the efficiency of the nursing process, allowing more time for direct patient care.
   b. Computers enhance the nurse-patient relationship by reinforcing the patient's belief that information will be kept confidential.
   c. Computers help make patient information legible.
   d. Computers help link diverse sources of patient information, broadening the horizons of nursing research and allowing for nursing decisions to be made on a more scientific basis.

9. All of the following are potential benefits of implementing a nationwide Nursing Minimum Data Set *except:*
   a. stimulation of nursing research through links to information stored in NISs.
   b. generation of data about nursing care that can be used to influence health policy decisions.
   c. instant consultation with nursing experts through an on-line bulletin board system.
   d. more accurate validation of the defining characteristics of nursing diagnoses.

10. The aim of those developing artificial intelligence is to create programs that:
    a. collect, display, and store data.
    b. simulate the human thinking process.
    c. enhance knowledge by providing large amounts of information quickly.
    d. provide a selection of standardized phrases for documentation.

(For answers with rationales, turn to page 265.)

FURTHER READINGS

Bleich, M.R., and Burton, M.J. *Information Management and Computers*. Nurse Managers' Bookshelf Series. Baltimore: Williams & Wilkins Co., 1990.

Brady, M. "Bedside Nursing/Hospital Information System Integration Must Include Productivity Gains for Nursing," *Computers in Nursing* 9(4):134-38, July-August 1991.

Brennan, P.F., and Romano, C.A. "Computers and Nursing Diagnosis: Issues in Implementation," *Nursing Clinics of North America* 22(4):935-41, December 1987.

Downing, D., and Covington, M. *Dictionary of Computer Terms*. New York: Barron's Educational Services, Inc., 1986.

Faaso, N. "Automated Patient Care Systems: The Ethical Impact," *Nursing Management* 23(7):46-48, July 1992.

Ford, J. "Computers and Nursing: Possibilities for Transforming Nursing," *Computers in Nursing* 8(4):160-64, July/August 1990.

Gordon, B., and Braun, D. "Automating a Clinical Management System," *Caring* 9(6):40-43, June 1990.

Hard, R. "Getting Nurses to Adopt Patient Care Computers," *Hospitals* 66(12):58, 60, June 20, 1992.

"Jargonese: A Guide to the Language of Computers," *Nursing Times* 85(29):72, July 19-25, 1989.

Lower, M.S., and Nauert, L.B. "Charting: The Impact of Bedside Computers," *Nursing Management* 23(7):40-42, 44, July 1992.

McHugh, M. "Computer Support for the Nursing Process," *Health Matrix* 7(1):57-60, Spring 1989.

Meintz, S.L., and Shaha, S.H. "Our Hand-held Computer Beats Them All," *RN* 55(1):52-55, 57, January 1992.

Meyer, C. "Bedside Computer Charting: Inching Toward Tomorrow," *American Journal of Nursing* 92(4):38-44, April 1992.

Miller, L.P. "Nursing, Computers, and Quality Care," *Med-Surg Quarterly* 1(3):104-18, Winter 1992.

Page-Greifinger, L. "Saving Time with a Computer," *Caring* 9(6):52-54, June 1990.

Perry, W.F., and Mornhinweg, G.C. "Nursing Practice: Promoting Computer Literacy," *Nursing Management* 23(7):49-52, July 1992.

Ponder, P.M. "The Nursing Process and Computers," *Point of View/Ethicon* 27(1):14-15, January 1, 1990.

Ripich, S., et al. "The New Nursing Medium: Computer Networks for Group Intervention," *Journal of Psychosocial Nursing and Mental Health Services* 30(7):15-20, July 1992.

Romano, C.A. "Privacy, Confidentiality, and Security of Computerized Systems: The Nursing Responsibility," *Computers in Nursing* 5(3):99-104, May-June 1987.

Schlehofer, G.B. "Informatics: Managing Clinical Operations Data," *Nursing Management* 23(7):36-38, July 1992.

Schmaus, D.C. "Choosing the Right System: Communicating Between Mainframe and Personal Computers," *AORN Journal* 51(1):236-39, January 1990.

Werley, H.H., and Zorn, C.R. "The Nursing Minimum Data Set and Its Relationship to Classifications for Nursing Practice," in *Classification Systems for Describing Nursing Practice*. Kansas City, Mo.: American Nurses' Association, 1989.

APPENDICES AND INDEX

QUICK REFERENCE TO NURSING DIAGNOSES

NURSING DIAGNOSIS AND DEFINITION	ASSOCIATED ASSESSMENT FINDINGS
Activity intolerance Inability to perform simple activities (such as activities of daily living) because of insufficient physical or psychological energy	• Dyspnea with activity • Activity interrupted frequently because of breathlessness or pain • Reports of fatigue or weakness
Activity intolerance, high risk for Accentuated risk of being unable to perform simple activities; danger that internal energy resources will not be sufficient to meet energy needs	• History of activity intolerance • Poor nutrition • Sleep deprivation • High metabolic needs (possibly caused by fever, large wounds, restlessness, or agitation)
Adjustment, impaired Inability to adjust behavior or lifestyle to compensate for changes in health status	• Expressions of shock, anger, and disbelief related to a change in health or ability to perform usual role • Reluctance to participate in planning for health status change • Inability to adhere to treatment plan
Airway clearance, ineffective Presence of anatomic or physiologic airway obstruction that impedes ventilation	• "Rattling" respirations • Weak or absent cough • Tenacious or copious secretions • Decreased level of consciousness • Diminished or absent gag reflex
Anxiety Feeling of apprehension or uneasiness without an identifiable cause	• Expressions of feeling tense, unsettled, and nervous • Irritability • Restlessness • Crying • Dry mouth • Tremulous voice • Increased heart and respiratory rates
Aspiration, high risk for Susceptibility to the passage of GI fluids, oral secretions, food, or fluids into the tracheobronchial tree	• Weak or absent cough • Weak or absent gag reflex • Decreased gastric emptying • Large gastric residuals • Wired jaws • Enteral feeding tube (especially small bore), endotracheal tube, or tracheostomy

QUICK REFERENCE TO NURSING DIAGNOSES – *continued*

NURSING DIAGNOSIS AND DEFINITION	ASSOCIATED ASSESSMENT FINDINGS
Body image disturbance Negative feelings toward self caused by changes in the body's appearance or function	• Loss of a body part • Refusal to look at or touch own body • Attempt to conceal a body part • Expression by patient of fear of being rejected because of altered body appearance or function
Body temperature, altered: High risk for Accentuated risk of failure to maintain body temperature within normal range	• Extremes of age: prematurity or old age • Emboli or cerebral bleeding in the brain stem • High metabolic rate (possibly caused by agitation, fever, shivering, or repeated generalized tonic-clonic seizures) • Exposure to hot or cold environmental temperatures • Illness or trauma affecting temperature regulation
Bowel incontinence Involuntary, uncontrolled passage of stools	• Involuntary defecation • Poor rectal sphincter control • Neurologic conditions resulting in the loss of sensation in the bowel
Breast-feeding, effective Satisfaction with the breast-feeding experience, with infant receiving adequate nutrition	• Mother expresses satisfaction with breast-feeding. • Infant is content after feedings. • Mother helps infant latch onto breast and suckle. • Mother demonstrates understanding of breast care. • Mother can interpret infant's cues to continue or discontinue feeding.
Breast-feeding, ineffective Dissatisfaction with breast-feeding on the part of the mother or neonate; difficulty with the breast-feeding process	• Actual or perceived inadequate milk supply • Neonate unable to latch onto the breast or sustain suckling • Neonatal weight loss • Retracted nipples • Neonate fussy and discontented after feedings
Breast-feeding, interrupted Interruption in the breast-feeding process caused by maternal or neonatal problem	• Neonate fails to receive sufficient nourishment for some or all feedings. • Mother expresses continued desire to maintain lactation and provide breast milk for neonate's nutritional needs.

(continued)

QUICK REFERENCE TO NURSING DIAGNOSES – *continued*

NURSING DIAGNOSIS AND DEFINITION	ASSOCIATED ASSESSMENT FINDINGS
Breathing pattern, ineffective State in which attempts to inhale and exhale fail to provide adequate gas exchange	• Nasal flaring • Accessory muscle use • Pursed-lip breathing • Reluctance to breathe deeply because of pain • Bradypnea, orthopnea, tachypnea, or periodic apnea • Splinting or guarding of the chest or abdominal muscles
Caregiver role strain Difficulty and stress experienced when seeking to meet the demands of being the family caregiver	• Caregiver reports not having adequate resources to provide the care needed (time, emotional strength, or physical energy). • Caregiver expresses worry about the care recipient's health and emotional state. • Caregiver reports difficulty performing other important roles (career, family, social) because of caregiving responsibilities. • Caregiver expresses feelings of loss because care recipient has changed. • Caregiver describes feeling stress or anxiety in relationship with care recipient.
Caregiver role strain, high risk for State in which caregiver is vulnerable to experiencing difficulty in performing the family caregiver role	• Care recipient has significant home care needs. • Caregiver is ill or elderly. • Caregiver is developmentally unprepared to provide care. • Caregiver has marginal coping patterns. • Care recipient will need care for a long time. • Caregiver has competing role requirements.
Communication, impaired verbal Decreased or absent ability to use or understand language to express needs or feelings	• Inability to speak dominant language • Slurred or garbled speech • Impaired articulation • Embolism or cerebral bleeding that interferes with speech center • Stuttering • Weak or absent voice • Hearing deficit

QUICK REFERENCE TO NURSING DIAGNOSES – *continued*

NURSING DIAGNOSIS AND DEFINITION	ASSOCIATED ASSESSMENT FINDINGS
Constipation Change in bowel habits character-ized by reduced frequency of stools and hard, dry stools	• Abdominal distention • Feeling of abdominal bloating • Nausea • Change in appetite • Infrequent, hard, dry stools • Straining during defecation • Inadequate fiber and fluid intake • Decreased activity level • Use of constipating medications
Constipation, colonic Elimination pattern characterized by hard, dry stools resulting from delayed passage of food residue	• Infrequent, hard, dry stools • Abdominal distention • Reports by patient of feeling rectal pressure and the need to strain when defecating • Inadequate fluid and fiber intake • Use of constipating medications • Fecal impaction
Constipation, perceived State in which an individual makes a self-diagnosis of consti-pation and uses laxatives, ene-mas, or suppositories to ensure a daily bowel movement	• Expectation that bowel movement should occur daily at a specific time • Long-term use of laxatives, enemas, or suppositories • Inability to move bowels without using laxatives
Decisional conflict State of uncertainty about which option to choose because of feared loss or challenge to per-sonal values	• Reports of uncertainty about choices • Delays in decision making • Expression of concern about the consequences of making a wrong choice • Signs of physical distress (increased pulse rate, restless-ness, anxiety) • Numerous requests for opinions about decision
Decreased cardiac output State in which the heart's pump-ing action is insufficient to meet the body's need for blood and oxygen	• Variations in blood pressure levels • Arrhythmias • Jugular vein distention • Decreased peripheral pulses • Cold, clammy skin • Mucous membrane and skin color changes • Oliguria • Dyspnea, orthopnea, crackles • Fatigue, restlessness

(continued)

QUICK REFERENCE TO NURSING DIAGNOSES – *continued*

NURSING DIAGNOSIS AND DEFINITION	ASSOCIATED ASSESSMENT FINDINGS
Defensive coping Falsely positive self-evaluation rooted in the need to protect against perceived threats to a positive self-image	• Denial of problems or difficulties obvious to others • Blaming own failures or weaknesses on others • Rationalization of inability to complete tasks successfully • Hypersensitivity to criticism
Denial, ineffective Conscious or unconscious attempt to deny the meaning of an event to decrease fear (This denial is detrimental to health.)	• Prolonged delay in seeking attention for serious illness or injury • Refusal to seek health care • Attempts to minimize discomfort • Attempts to attribute symptom to another source (for example, saying that chest pain is caused by anxiety or indigestion when it is really caused by angina)
Diarrhea Change in normal bowel pattern characterized by liquid, unformed stools	• Frequent loose stools • Increased flatus • Hyperactive bowel sounds • Abdominal cramps or pain • Rectal urgency • Perianal tenderness
Disuse syndrome, high risk for State of being at risk for deterioration of a body part as a result of prescribed or unavoidable inactivity	• Flaccid or spastic paralysis • Muscle wasting • Decreased level of consciousness • Severe pain • Prolonged immobilization from traction, casts, or bed rest
Diversional activity deficit Restriction or decrease in ability to use unoccupied time to advantage or satisfaction	• Expression of boredom • Long-term hospitalization • Frequent extensive treatments • Physical limitations that affect ability to participate in usual activities or hobbies
Dysreflexia State in which a patient with a spinal cord injury (T7 or higher) experiences a severe sympathetic nervous system response to a painful or unpleasant stimulus	• Sudden, severely elevated blood pressure • Increased or decreased heart rate • Diaphoresis and red splotches above the level of the spinal cord injury • Pallor below the level of the spinal cord injury • Headache • Bladder distention • Abdominal distention

QUICK REFERENCE TO NURSING DIAGNOSES – *continued*

NURSING DIAGNOSIS AND DEFINITION	ASSOCIATED ASSESSMENT FINDINGS
Family coping, ineffective: Compromised Behavior of family members that compromises the patient's and family's capacity to adapt	• Family members withdraw from patient or are preoccupied with their own reaction to the change in the patient's health status. • Patient expresses concerns about family members' responses to health problem. • Family members express an inadequate understanding of the patient's health problem, which interferes with their ability to support or assist patient.
Family coping, ineffective: Disabling Behavior of family members that undermines the patient's and family's ability to adapt	• Family members deny existence or severity of patient's health problem. • Family members go about usual routine without regard for the patient's needs. • Family members' decisions and actions are detrimental to economic or social well-being. • Family members neglect each other's needs. • Patient develops helpless, dependent attitude.
Family coping: Potential for growth Demonstrated ability of a family member to cope effectively with the patient's changed health status accompanied by an expression of a desire to improve health, personal growth, and relationship to the patient	• Family member describes the impact that health crisis has had on personal values, goals, and relationships. • Family member expresses an interest in health promotion activities and support groups. • Family member assists in making decisions related to patient's treatment options.
Family process, altered State in which normally functional family is unable to act effectively when experiencing a crisis	• Family system unable to meet physical, emotional, and spiritual needs of its members. • Family members fail to respect each other's individuality and autonomy. • Family members refuse to accept help. • Family members are unable to accept or express a wide range of feelings. • Family members are unable to adjust to change or deal with trauma. • Family members fail to communicate effectively. • Parents do not respect each other's child-rearing views.

(continued)

QUICK REFERENCE TO NURSING DIAGNOSES – *continued*

NURSING DIAGNOSIS AND DEFINITION	ASSOCIATED ASSESSMENT FINDINGS
Fatigue An overwhelming feeling of exhaustion and decreased capacity to perform physical and mental labor	• Reports by patient of continual, unrelieved lack of energy • Inability to perform activities of daily living • Inability to concentrate • Tendency to be accident-prone • Apathy, irritability, lethargy
Fear Feeling of dread or impending disaster related to an identifiable source	• Identifiable fear-producing situation • Experience of loss of control reported by patient • Tremulous voice • Increased respiratory rate • Limb tremors
Fluid volume deficit Excessive loss of vascular, cellular, or extracellular fluid	• Change in urine output, urine concentration, and serum sodium levels • Sudden weight loss or gain • Decreased venous filling • Hemoconcentration • Hypotension • Thirst • Increased body temperature and pulse rate • Dry mucous membranes and skin • Mental status change • Weakness
Fluid volume deficit, high risk for State in which patient is susceptible to excessive vascular, cellular, and extracellular fluid loss	• Increased metabolic demands caused by fever or restlessness • Diarrhea • Vomiting • Draining wounds • GI sectioning • Administration of diuretics • Extremes of age: very young or very old patient
Fluid volume excess State in which patient experiences increased fluid retention and edema	• Edema • Weight gain • Shortness of breath • Orthopnea • Fluid intake that exceeds output • Oliguria • Chest auscultation reveals S_3 heart sound and crackles • Neck vein distention • Anxiety and restlessness

QUICK REFERENCE TO NURSING DIAGNOSES – *continued*

NURSING DIAGNOSIS AND DEFINITION	ASSOCIATED ASSESSMENT FINDINGS
Gas exchange, impaired Interference in the ability to exchange carbon dioxide and oxygen between the alveoli and the pulmonary vascular bed	• Shortness of breath • Confusion • Irritability • Restlessness • Somnolence • Inability to move secretions • Hyperpnea • Hypoxia
Grieving, anticipatory Grief response that results from perception that loss of someone or something valued is imminent	• Impending divorce or separation • Terminal illness of patient • Serious illness of family member or friend • Decreased ability to perform daily roles • Need to relocate to another area • Financial problems • Expressions of anger, sorrow, or guilt • Expressions of distress at potential loss
Grieving, dysfunctional Inability to move through the stages of the grief process after an actual or perceived loss	• Verbalization of distress at loss • Denial of loss • Expression of guilt or unresolved issues related to the loss • Displays of anger, sadness, or crying • Inability to concentrate • Changes in eating and sleeping habits • Altered libido • Reluctance to accept help to work through the loss
Growth and development, altered Deviation in growth and development compared with norms for age-group	• Delay or difficulty in developing motor, social, or verbal skills appropriate for age-group • Physical growth changes • Inability to perform self-care activities or exhibit level of self-control appropriate for age-group • Flat affect, listlessness, and decreased response to environmental stimuli
Health maintenance, altered Inability to identify and manage health care problems and to obtain resources for meeting health care needs	• Lack of knowledge about health care practices • Inadequate financial resources to meet health care needs • Inadequate social support systems • Inability to make sound judgments regarding self-care because of cognitive impairment • Inability to care for self because of lack of motor skills

(continued)

QUICK REFERENCE TO NURSING DIAGNOSES – *continued*

NURSING DIAGNOSIS AND DEFINITION	ASSOCIATED ASSESSMENT FINDINGS
Health-seeking behaviors State in which a patient in stable health actively pursues ways to change personal health habits and the environment to improve health status	• Expressed desire to pursue a higher level of wellness • Unfamiliarity with community wellness resources • Lack of knowledge about health-promoting behaviors
Home maintenance management, impaired Inability to maintain a home environment that promotes safety, health, or personal growth	• Unwashed clothing and cooking equipment • Absence of heat and running water • Infestation by vermin and rodents • Family members' reports of feeling exhausted • Family members' expressions of difficulty maintaining their home and requests for assistance • Family members' reports of inadequate financial resources
Hopelessness Inability to perceive personal options or use available resources for improvement	• Decreased verbalization • Flat affect • Passivity • Expressions of being unable to change situation • Changes in appetite and sleep pattern • Sighs, shrugs, and failure to maintain eye contact • Apathy toward care • Verbal expressions of hopelessness
Hyperthermia Elevation of body temperature above normal range	• Fever • Flushed and warm skin • Increased pulse and respiratory rates • Decreased skin turgor
Hypothermia Decrease in body temperature below normal range	• Cool skin • Shivering • Piloerection • Pallor • Cyanotic nail beds • Rapid pulse rate • Hypertension
Incontinence, functional Inability to control or predict the excretion of urine	• Involuntary loss of urine • Failure to recognize warning signs of bladder fullness • Voiding that occurs in socially unacceptable situations

QUICK REFERENCE TO NURSING DIAGNOSES – *continued*

NURSING DIAGNOSIS AND DEFINITION	ASSOCIATED ASSESSMENT FINDINGS
Incontinence, reflex Involuntary loss of urine occurring at predictable intervals when the bladder fills to a specific volume	• Lack of awareness of bladder filling • Lack of urge to void or feelings of bladder fullness • Bladder contraction or spasm occurring at regular intervals
Incontinence, stress Involuntary loss of less than 50 ml of urine that occurs with increased intra-abdominal pressure	• Urine dribbling with increased intra-abdominal pressure (such as when coughing, laughing, or sneezing) • Urinary frequency and urgency
Incontinence, total Continuous and unpredictable involuntary loss of urine	• Steady flow of urine without bladder distention, contraction, or spasm • Patient unaware of full bladder or incontinence
Incontinence, urge Involuntary loss of urine shortly after the urge to urinate	• Urgency and frequency • Bladder contraction and spasm • Inability to reach toilet or bedpan in time • Small amount (less than 100 ml) or large amount (more than 550 ml) of urine excreted at each voiding • Nocturia
Individual coping, ineffective Diminished ability to adapt to life's demands or to solve problems	• Expression by patient of inability to cope or to find help • Difficulty solving problems • Behavior that is destructive toward self or others • Changes in social habits • Inappropriate use of defense mechanisms • Change in communication patterns
Infant feeding pattern, ineffective Impaired ability of infant to suck or to coordinate the suck-swallow response	• Inability of infant to initiate or sustain effective sucking • Inability of infant to coordinate sucking, swallowing, and breathing
Infection, high risk for Increased risk of invasion by pathogenic organisms or diminished ability to defend against invasion by pathogenic organisms	• Broken skin or mucous membranes • Stasis of body fluids • Multiple invasive lines or procedures • Administration of immunosuppressant drugs • Diminished nutritional status • Inadequate understanding of infection prevention measures

(continued)

QUICK REFERENCE TO NURSING DIAGNOSES *– continued*

NURSING DIAGNOSIS AND DEFINITION	ASSOCIATED ASSESSMENT FINDINGS
Injury, high risk for Accentuated risk of physical harm from dangers in environment	• Altered balance or gait • Impaired judgment • Confusion • Weakness • Unsafe physical environment
Knowledge deficit Inadequate understanding of information or inability to perform skills needed to practice health-related behaviors	• Lack of exposure • Lack of recall • Poor cognitive abilities • Disinterest in learning • Unfamiliarity with relevant information
Management of therapeutic regimen, ineffective Inability to integrate program for treating illness and its effects into daily life	• Inappropriate choices with regard to meeting goals of treatment or prevention program • Exacerbation of symptoms • Reports by patient of difficulty with health care regimen
Noncompliance Unwillingness to follow recommended treatment plan	• Failure of patient to adhere to prescribed treatments, such as diet, medications, and mobility restrictions • Development of complications • Exacerbation of symptoms • Failure of patient to progress or keep appointments • Inability of patient and caregivers to establish and maintain mutual goals
Nutrition, altered: High risk for more than body requirements State in which a patient is at risk for experiencing an intake of nutrients that exceeds metabolic needs	• Dysfunctional eating habits, such as eating in response to internal cues other than hunger or concentrating intake at end of day • Sedentary life-style • History of obesity • Immobility • Excessive preoccupation with food

QUICK REFERENCE TO NURSING DIAGNOSES – *continued*

NURSING DIAGNOSIS AND DEFINITION	ASSOCIATED ASSESSMENT FINDINGS
Nutrition, altered: Less than body requirements Nutritional intake that is insufficient to meet metabolic needs and that results in unhealthful weight loss	• Weight at least 20% less than ideal for patient • Weakening of muscles used for chewing and swallowing • Lack of interest in food • Perceived inability to eat food • Reports by patient of altered sense of taste and abdominal cramping • Hyperactive bowel sounds • Inadequate muscle tone • Pale conjunctiva and mucous membranes • Excessive hair loss
Nutrition, altered: More than body requirements Excessive nutritional intake and increased body weight resulting from change in eating pattern	• Body weight 10% or more over ideal • Triceps skinfold thickness more than 15 mm in male patients and more than 25 mm in female patients • Dysfunctional eating habits (eating in response to internal cues other than hunger) • Sedentary life-style
Oral mucous membrane, altered Altered mouth integrity	• Carious teeth • Coated tongue • Decreased or absent salivation • Desquamation • Dry mouth • Gum hypertrophy or recession • Halitosis • Hyperemia • Inflammation of gums or mucous membranes • Leukoplakia • Oral edema, bleeding, or exudate • Oral lesions, vesicles, or ulcers • Oral pain or discomfort • Oral plaque
Pain Subjective sensation of discomfort that may result from physical, chemical, biological, or psychological stimuli	• Guarding or protective behavior, such as favoring an affected body part • Facial mask of pain, characterized by lackluster eyes, a "beaten" look, fixed or scattered movement, or grimacing • Crying or moaning • Verbal reports of pain • Restlessness • Changes in blood pressure, pulse rate, and respiratory rate

(continued)

QUICK REFERENCE TO NURSING DIAGNOSES – *continued*

NURSING DIAGNOSIS AND DEFINITION	ASSOCIATED ASSESSMENT FINDINGS
Pain, chronic Subjective sensation of discomfort that is unrelieved for 6 months or more	• Verbal reports of chronic pain • Guarded movements • Changes in sleep patterns or activity levels • Reluctance to maintain activities • Withdrawal • Attitude of discouragement • Depression related to unrelieved pain • Fatigue • Decreased perception and awareness of surroundings
Parental role conflict State in which one or both parents experience confusion and conflict during a crisis	• Expression by parents of feeling inadequate to meet the child's needs • Expression by parents of concern about changes in their role and alterations in family functioning, communication, and health • Ineffective parental coping mechanisms
Parenting, altered Inability of a parent or nurturing figure to create an environment that fosters growth and development of an infant or a child	• Indifference to the child's needs • Lack of attachment behaviors on the part of the parent (eye contact, calling the child by name, or speaking to the child) • Unsuitable caregiving behavior (feeding or toilet training) • Parental history of abandonment or child abuse • Verbalization of resentment toward the child
Parenting, altered: High risk for Presence of risk factors that may interfere with parents' ability to create an environment that promotes optimal growth and development of an infant or a child	• Lack of role model for parents • Insufficient support available to parents • Frequent injuries or illnesses in the infant or child • Inappropriate or inconsistent discipline • Lack of knowledge about appropriate parenting behaviors
Peripheral neurovascular dysfunction, high risk for Accentuated risk of disrupted circulation, sensation, or motion in an extremity	• Fracture • Mechanical compression (tourniquet, cast, brace, dressing, or restraint) • Orthopedic surgery • Trauma • Immobilization • Burns • Vascular obstruction

QUICK REFERENCE TO NURSING DIAGNOSES – *continued*

NURSING DIAGNOSIS AND DEFINITION	ASSOCIATED ASSESSMENT FINDINGS
Personal identity disturbance Inability to differentiate between self and nonself	• Agitation, disorientation, hallucinations • Increased sensitivity to environmental stimuli • Objects and events in environment take on undue personal significance
Physical mobility, impaired Limited ability to move independently	• Inability to move purposely within the environment • Hesitancy to attempt to move • Limited range of motion • Reduced muscle strength
Poisoning, high risk for Accentuated risk of accidental exposure to or ingestion of drugs or other dangerous substances in amounts sufficient to result in poisoning	• Decreased vision • Cognitive impairment • Unsafe environment (for example, hazardous working conditions or unsecured medicine cabinet) • Presence of flaking lead-base paint in the home
Posttrauma response Sustained painful response to a traumatic event	• Reexperience of trauma • Hyperalertness • Flashbacks • Nightmares • Frequent verbalization about the event • Feelings of guilt related to surviving the event
Powerlessness Perception that one's personal actions will have little effect on the outcome of a situation	• Expressions by patient indicating lack of control over self or environment • Depression • Apathy • Lack of participation in health care activities or decision making • Fear and passivity • Dependence on others
Protection, altered Reduced ability to protect self from illness or injury	• Anorexia • Chills • Cough, dyspnea • Perspiration, itching • Immobility, fatigue, weakness • Restlessness, insomnia, disorientation • Pressure ulcers • Impaired clotting mechanism • Deficient immunity

(continued)

QUICK REFERENCE TO NURSING DIAGNOSES – *continued*

NURSING DIAGNOSIS AND DEFINITION	ASSOCIATED ASSESSMENT FINDINGS
Rape-trauma syndrome Physical and emotional trauma that occurs as a result of sexual assault	• Expressions of anger, embarrassment, and humiliation • Fear of physical violence and death • Self-blame • Expression of desire for revenge • GI disturbances • Genitourinary discomfort • Increased muscle tension • Sleep pattern changes
Rape-trauma syndrome: Compound reaction Trauma syndrome that develops after rape or attempted rape in which the patient experiences drastic changes in behavior, psychological equilibrium, and ability to function	• Acute phase: anger, embarrassment, humiliation, fear of physical violence and death, revenge seeking, self-blame, hysterical outbursts, homicidal ideation, suicidal ideation, multiple physical symptoms (GI disturbances, genitourinary discomfort, increased muscle tension, sleep pattern changes), renewed symptoms of previous physical or psychiatric illness, dependence on alcohol or drugs • Long-term phase: changes in life-style, including change of residence, seeking support from family and social network, repetitive nightmares
Rape-trauma syndrome: Silent reaction Trauma syndrome that develops after rape or attempted rape in which the patient doesn't tell anyone about the rape or deal with her feelings about it	• Abrupt changes in relationships with the opposite sex • Increased anxiety during interview • Increased nightmares • No verbal indication that rape occurred • Pronounced changes in sexual behavior • Sudden onset of phobic reactions • Signs and symptoms of posttraumatic response
Relocation stress syndrome Physiologic or psychological disturbance caused by a move to a new environment	• Anxiety • Apprehension • Increased confusion (especially among elderly patients) • Depression • Loneliness • Expression of dissatisfaction with relocation • Change in eating patterns • Withdrawal

QUICK REFERENCE TO NURSING DIAGNOSES – *continued*

NURSING DIAGNOSIS AND DEFINITION	ASSOCIATED ASSESSMENT FINDINGS
Role performance, altered Disruption in the ability to perform usual social, vocational, or family roles	• Altered perception of role • Denial of role or responsibility • Conflict between roles • Change in physical capacity to resume role • Misunderstanding of demands of role • Recent change in usual pattern or level of responsibility
Self-care deficit: Bathing and hygiene Inability to bathe independently or to perform hygienic measures	• Inability to wash body or body parts • Inability to get to water source or acquire bath supplies • Inability to control water temperature or flow
Self-care deficit: Dressing and grooming Inability to dress independently or to perform grooming measures	• Inability to put on or take off clothing • Impaired ability to obtain or replace articles of clothing • Inability to fasten clothing • Inability to maintain satisfactory appearance
Self-care deficit: Feeding Inability to feed self	• Inability to bring food from receptacle to mouth
Self-care deficit: Toileting Inability to carry out toileting routine	• Inability to walk to toilet or commode • Inability to sit on toilet or commode • Inability to remove clothing for toileting • Inability to flush toilet or empty commode • Inability to carry out proper toilet hygiene
Self-esteem, chronic low A long-standing negative appraisal of self or capabilities	• Expression of negative feelings about self or abilities • Reluctance to try new options • Rejection of positive feedback about self from others • Expression of doubt about ability to deal with challenges or new situations • Lack of success in or mastery of life situations
Self-esteem, situational low Development of negative feelings about self after a change or loss	• Expression of negative feelings about self, such as helplessness and uselessness, in response to life events in a person with a previously positive self-evaluation • Expression of shame and guilt • Expression of feeling unable to affect the outcome of a situation • Difficulty making a decision

(continued)

QUICK REFERENCE TO NURSING DIAGNOSES – *continued*

NURSING DIAGNOSIS AND DEFINITION	ASSOCIATED ASSESSMENT FINDINGS
Self-esteem disturbance Negative feelings about self or capabilities that may be directly or indirectly expressed	• Verbalization of self-negating thoughts • Expression of shame and guilt • Evaluation of self as unable to cope with events • Reluctance to participate in new situations • Denial of problems that are obvious to others • Hypersensitivity to slights or criticism • Displays of grandiosity
Self-mutilation, high risk for State in which an individual is at risk for performing a deliberate act of self-harm that's intended to produce immediate tissue damage	• Lability of affect • Borderline personality disorder • Psychotic state • Childhood emotional disturbances or abuse • Expressions of self-hatred • Feelings of depression or emptiness • History of dysfunctional family upbringing • Inability to cope with increased stress • Lack of self-esteem • History of self-injury

Sensory or perceptual alterations (visual, auditory, kinesthetic, gustatory, tactile, olfactory)
Diminished or altered ability to interpret incoming sensory stimuli
	• Disorientation to person, place, and time
	• Reported alterations in sensory acuity
	  — Evidence of decreased hearing ability
	  — Altered sense of smell or taste, weight loss, loss of appetite
	  — Altered kinesthetic sense: diminished motor coordination; inability to identify location of body part; inability to perceive changes in angles of joints; muscle weakness, flaccidity, rigidity, or atrophy; paralysis
	  — Evidence of impaired visual ability or visual distortions
	• Altered communication patterns
	• Altered conceptualization
	• Change in usual response to stimuli
	• Anxiety
	• Apathy
	• Irritability
	• Restlessness
	• Depression
	• Hallucinations

QUICK REFERENCE TO NURSING DIAGNOSES – *continued*

NURSING DIAGNOSIS AND DEFINITION	ASSOCIATED ASSESSMENT FINDINGS
Sexual dysfunction Alteration in one's usual pattern of sexual function because of physical or emotional factors	• Expression of dissatisfaction with current level of sexual functioning • Actual or perceived sexual limitation caused by illness or treatment • Seeking affirmation of desirability • Change in relationship with spouse or significant other • Decreased level of interest in self and others
Sexuality patterns, altered State in which an individual expresses concern about personal sexuality	• Reports of alterations, difficulties, or limitations in sexual activities • Emotional and behavioral reactions, including anger, constricted affect, depressed mood, noncompliance with prescribed therapies, and withdrawal from social interaction
Skin integrity, impaired Interruption in skin integrity	• Disruption of skin surfaces • Destruction of skin layers • Invasion of body structures • Clinical evidence of internal factors that adversely affect skin integrity (for example, altered nutritional status, dermatologic conditions, or loss of subcutaneous tissue or muscle mass) • Clinical evidence of external factors that adversely affect skin integrity (for example, chemical agents, cold, heat, or pressure)
Skin integrity, impaired: High risk for Accentuated risk of interruption or destruction of skin surface	• Pressure, friction, or shearing forces • Restraints • Excretions and secretions • Confinement to bed or chair • Decreased serum albumin levels • Dependence on others for self-care • Bowel or bladder incontinence • Decreased circulation • Obesity • Localized infection in pressure-supporting areas • Loss of subcutaneous tissue or muscle mass • Physical immobility • Change in nutritional status • Comatose state • Skin maceration • Dehydration

(continued)

QUICK REFERENCE TO NURSING DIAGNOSES – *continued*

NURSING DIAGNOSIS AND DEFINITION	ASSOCIATED ASSESSMENT FINDINGS
Sleep pattern disturbance Disruption in the ability to meet individual need for sleep or rest	• Report by patient of difficulty falling asleep, awakening earlier or later than wanted, or interrupted sleep • Altered behaviors: disorientation, irritability, lethargy, listlessness, or restlessness • Physical changes: dark circles under eyes, expressionless face, frequent yawning, posture changes
Social interaction, impaired Dissatisfaction with the quality or quantity of social contacts and interactions	• Reports by patient of discomfort in social situations • Observations of dysfunctional social interaction patterns • Inability to receive or communicate a sense of belonging and sharing
Social isolation Aloneness that is perceived negatively by the patient and which may be self-imposed, perceived to be imposed by others, or the result of environmental factors	• Lack of support from family and friends • Verbalization of feelings of aloneness and rejection • Inappropriate activities or interests in relation to developmental age • Hostility projected in voice and behavior • Evidence of physical or mental disability • Failure to maintain eye contact • Uncommunicative, withdrawn demeanor
Spiritual distress Separation or alienation from religious tradition or spiritual values	• Questioning of the meaning of life • Expression of anger toward God • Refusal to participate in usual religious practices • Expressions of concern about ethical and moral ramifications of treatment • Mood changes: anger, anxiety, apathy, crying, hostility, withdrawal • Expression of inner conflicts
Spontaneous ventilation, inability to sustain Inability to sustain breathing sufficient to support life	• Apprehension • Decreased cooperation • Decreased partial pressure of oxygen in arterial blood (PaO_2) • Decreased arterial oxygen saturation • Increased partial pressure of carbon dioxide in arterial blood ($PaCO_2$) • Dyspnea • Increased metabolic rate • Restlessness • Increased use of accessory muscles • Respiratory muscle fatigue • Tachycardia

QUICK REFERENCE TO NURSING DIAGNOSES – *continued*

NURSING DIAGNOSIS AND DEFINITION	ASSOCIATED ASSESSMENT FINDINGS
Suffocation, high risk for Accentuated risk of accidental suffocation (inadequate air available for inhalation)	• Diminished sense of smell • Impaired mobility • Improper positioning of immobile patient • Lack of safety education and precautions • Unsupervised children (for example, children inserting small objects into their mouths or noses or playing with plastic bags) • Smoking in bed • Consumption of large mouthfuls of food • Ventilator connections improperly monitored • Ventilator alarms turned off
Swallowing, impaired Reduced ability to move food or fluids from the mouth through the esophagus	• Choking or coughing when taking food or fluids • Stasis of food in oral cavity • Decreased or absent gag reflex • Evidence of aspiration • Facial paralysis
Thermoregulation, ineffective Fluctuations in body temperature caused by thermoregulatory disturbances	• Trauma or illness • Prematurity or old age • Fever or hypothermic condition refractory to antipyretic therapy • Flushed or mottled skin • Increased or decreased respiratory and heart rates • Mild to severe dehydration • Skin warm or cool to touch
Thought processes, altered Inability to process thoughts accurately and correctly	• Altered attention span • Clinical evidence of impaired neurologic or psychiatric functioning • Decreased ability to grasp ideas • Disorientation to time, place, person, circumstances, and events • Impaired ability to think abstractly or conceptualize • Impaired ability to calculate • Impaired ability to make decisions • Impaired ability to reason • Impaired ability to solve problems • Inability to follow instructions • Inappropriate social behavior • Memory deficit or problems

(continued)

QUICK REFERENCE TO NURSING DIAGNOSES – *continued*

NURSING DIAGNOSIS AND DEFINITION	ASSOCIATED ASSESSMENT FINDINGS
Tissue integrity, impaired Damage to mucous membranes or to corneal, integumentary, or subcutaneous tissue	• Damaged or destroyed tissue (cornea, mucous membranes, integumentary, or subcutaneous) • Altered circulation • Nutritional deficit or excess • Fluid deficit or excess • Impaired physical mobility • Peripheral vascular changes • Presence of chemical irritants (for example, body excretions) • Presence of mechanical irritants (for example, pressure or shearing forces) • Exposure to radiation • Blisters, blebs, edema, erythema, eschar, exudate, itching, odor, pain
Tissue perfusion, altered (renal, cerebral, cardiopulmonary, gastrointestinal, peripheral) Decrease in cellular nutrition and respiration caused by decreased capillary blood flow	• Renal: Abnormal serum electrolyte levels; dark, concentrated urine; decreased hemoglobin levels; decreased urine osmolality; decreased urine output; elevated blood urea nitrogen levels, serum creatinine levels, and creatinine clearance; increased blood pressure; peripheral edema; shortness of breath; weakness; weight gain • Cerebral: behavioral changes, change in level of consciousness, change in respiratory pattern, dizziness, dysphagia, eye deviation, headaches, impaired gag reflex, irritability, lethargy, memory loss, nausea and vomiting, orthostatic hypotension, photophobia, posturing, pupillary changes, restlessness, seizures, slurred speech, tinnitus, unilateral weakness or paralysis, visual changes • Cardiopulmonary: arrhythmias; electrocardiogram changes; abnormal arterial blood gas levels; chest pain with or without activity; cold, clammy skin; crackles; cyanosis; decreased peripheral pulses; elevated cardiac enzyme and isoenzyme levels; fatigue; hypotension; mental status changes; pallor of skin and mucous membranes; palpitations; edema; rhonchi; shortness of breath; slow capillary refill time; tachycardia; variations in hemodynamic readings • Gastrointestinal: absence of bowel sounds or change in their sound or frequency, abdominal pain associated with recently eaten meals, ascites or fluid wave,

QUICK REFERENCE TO NURSING DIAGNOSES – *continued*

NURSING DIAGNOSIS AND DEFINITION	ASSOCIATED ASSESSMENT FINDINGS
Tissue perfusion, altered *(continued)*	constipation, decrease in hematocrit and hemoglobin levels, diarrhea, history of recent abdominal surgery or blunt abdominal trauma, increase in white blood cell count or erythrocyte sedimentation rate, presence of occult blood, recent weight loss or gain, nausea, vomiting • Peripheral: anxiety; atrial arrhythmias; bruits; clinical evidence of interrupted or reduced arterial blood flow; decreased joint mobility; diminished or absent peripheral pulses; diminished sensitivity to pressure, temperature, or tissue trauma; edema of extremities; intermittent claudication; irritability; muscle wasting or weakness; numbness, tingling; obesity; skin changes (blanched when extremity is raised above level of heart, cool to touch, cyanotic with severe disease, gangrenous, glossy, hairless, pale, pruritic, slow-healing, trophic changes, ulcerated); trophic changes of nails
Trauma, high risk for Accentuated risk of accidental tissue injury, such as burns or fractures	• Balancing difficulties • Malnutrition • Poor vision • Reduced large- or small-muscle coordination • Reduced tactile sensation • Decreased body temperature • Weakness or fatigue • Bathtub lacking handgrip or antislip equipment • High bed • Inappropriate or broken call-for-aid mechanism for patient on bed rest • Litter or liquid spills on floor • Loose connections on invasive monitoring devices • Patient sliding on coarse bed linens or struggling with bed restraints • Unlighted rooms or corridors
Unilateral neglect Lack of awareness of a body part	• Denial of parts of the body affected by illness or trauma, either by refusing to acknowledge the body part, by neglecting the involved side, or by attributing ownership of a body part to someone else • Consistent inattention to stimuli on affected side • Inappropriate positioning of the affected side • Inadequate self-care • Neurologic illness or trauma • Hemianopsia

(continued)

QUICK REFERENCE TO NURSING DIAGNOSES – *continued*

NURSING DIAGNOSIS AND DEFINITION	ASSOCIATED ASSESSMENT FINDINGS
Urinary elimination pattern, altered Altered or impaired urinary function	• Dysuria and nocturia • Frequency, hesitancy, and urgency • Hematuria • Incontinence and retention • Clinical evidence of urinary obstruction or of sensory or neuromuscular impairment of urinary tract
Urinary retention Incomplete emptying of bladder	• Bladder distention • Dysuria and nocturia • Hesitancy • High level of residual urine • Loss of anal sphincter tone (with sensory or neuromuscular impairment) • Overflow incontinence (continuous dribbling) • Sensation of bladder fullness (possible) • Slow stream of urine • Small, frequent voidings or no urine output
Ventilatory weaning response, dysfunctional Difficulty adjusting to lowered levels of mechanical ventilator support, which interrupts and prolongs the weaning process	• Mild: breathing discomfort; expression of increased need for oxygen; fatigue; increased concentration on breathing; queries about possible machine malfunction; restlessness; warmth • Moderate: apprehension; changes in skin color, paleness, or slight cyanosis; decreased air entry on auscultation; inability to cooperate; inability to respond to coaching; blood pressure slightly increased (no more than 20 mm Hg above baseline), heart rate slightly increased (no more than 20 beats/minute above baseline), respiratory rate slightly increased (no more than 5 breaths/minute above baseline); slight accessory muscle use • Severe: adventitious breath sounds; agitation; audible airway secretions; cyanosis; decreased level of consciousness; deteriorating arterial blood gas levels; full respiratory accessory muscle use; elevated blood pressure (more than 20 mm Hg above baseline); increased heart rate (more than 20 beats/minute above baseline); respiratory rate increased significantly from baseline; paradoxical abdominal breathing; profuse diaphoresis; shallow, gasping breathing; breathing uncoordinated with ventilator

QUICK REFERENCE TO NURSING DIAGNOSES — *continued*

NURSING DIAGNOSIS AND DEFINITION	ASSOCIATED ASSESSMENT FINDINGS
Violence, high risk for: Self-directed or directed at others Presence of risk factors for suicide, assault, or other acts of violence	• Anger • Expressions of fear of self or others • History of assault, weapon possession, or arrest • Provocative behavior (argumentative, dissatisfied, hypersensitive, overreactive) • Impaired memory, judgment, and intellectual functioning • Inability to voice feelings • Increasing anxiety level • Increased motor activity, pacing, excitement, irritability, agitation • Overt and aggressive acts — goal-directed destruction of objects in environment • Self-destructive behavior and active, aggressive, suicidal acts • Suspicion of others, paranoid ideation, delusions, hallucinations • Direct or indirect statements indicating desire to kill oneself • Fear of own impulsivity • Feelings of helplessness, loneliness, hopelessness • History of previous suicide attempts • Substance abuse or withdrawal • Tense muscles • Vulnerable self-esteem

ANSWERS TO SELF-TEST QUESTIONS

Chapter 2: Assessment

1. **d.** The nursing health history is distinguished by its holistic focus on the human response to illness.

2. **a.** The three phases of the nursing health history interview are the introduction, body, and closure.

3. **b.** Subjective data represents the patient's perceptions; objective information can be observed and verified.

4. **d.** One appropriate interview technique is remaining silent for short periods to reduce anxiety and to give the patient a chance to organize his thoughts.

5. **a.** When trying to communicate with a hearing-impaired or an elderly patient, do not touch him to let him know you're in the room; you may startle him. Rather, when approaching the patient or entering his room, announce yourself. The other guidelines (making sure that the patient who wears eyeglasses has them on when you're speaking to him, beginning your talk by stating the subject of the conversation, and not rushing the patient when he is trying to express himself) are examples of appropriate measures of communicating with a hearing-impaired or an elderly patient.

6. **c.** When assessing a patient who speaks in an unfamiliar language or dialect, don't try to speak in his ethnic dialect to put him at ease; he may think you're mocking him or being condescending. The other guidelines (using titles such as "Mr." or "Mrs." unless you've established a first-name basis for the relationship, asking the patient's friend or family member to serve as a translator, and not assuming the patient is angry if he talks more loudly than is usual among Americans) are appropriate actions when assessing a patient who speaks an unfamiliar language or dialect.

7. **b.** An open-ended assessment form uses a "fill-in-the-blanks" style, and a closed-ended assessment form has checklists or questions with specific responses.

8. **d.** You obtain subjective information by listening to your patient's descriptions of his symptoms.

9. **b.** The primary source of assessment information is the patient.

10. **b.** The North American Nursing Diagnosis Association (NANDA) bases its classification system for nursing diagnoses on human response patterns.

11. **d.** When deciding on a method of physical examination, consider whether the patient's condition is life-threatening and the characteristics of your patient population, and try to use the same examination routine all of the time.

Chapter 3: Nursing diagnosis

1. **c.** A nursing diagnosis is a clinical judgment about human responses to health problems or life processes.

2. **e.** Unlike a medical diagnosis, a nursing diagnosis may change as the patient's responses change, may apply to the patient and his family, and focuses on the patient's perception of his health status as well as on his physical condition. Also, formulating a nursing diagnosis is within the legally permissible scope of nursing practice; a medical diagnosis, within the legally permissible scope of medical practice.

3. **a.** The NANDA taxonomy organizes nursing diagnoses under categories called human response patterns.

4. **e.** Moving, choosing, relating, and valuing are human response patterns; sharing is not.

5. **d.** The components to be included when developing a nursing diagnosis are the diagnostic label with qualifier, defining characteristics, and etiology.

6. **d.** In the statement *pain related to myocardial infarction,* the etiology is a medical diagnosis.

7. **c.** The statement *impaired home maintenance management related to laziness and lack of effort* reflects an inappropriate value judgment.

8. **a.** The nursing diagnosis statement *ineffective individual coping related to lack of social support* is correct as written.

9. **b.** In the statement *anger related to death of spouse,* the diagnostic label identifies an appropriate emotional response as unhealthful.

10. **b.** In the statement *daily tracheostomy care related to mucus buildup,* the diagnostic label identifies a nursing treatment instead of a patient problem.

Chapter 4: Planning

1. **d.** The plan of care includes the patient's nursing diagnoses, expected outcomes, nursing interventions, the patient-teaching plan, and evaluation data.

2. **d.** All caregivers, plus the patient and family members, should have access to the plan of care.

3. **b.** When setting care priorities, assign the highest priority to life-threatening problems and the lowest priority to needs that are not related to the patient's specific illness or prognosis.

4. **d.** Maslow's hierarchy of needs describes five levels of human needs and stresses that basic physiologic needs must be met before higher-level needs can be addressed.

5. **b.** According to Orem's self-care theory, the nurse's major goal is to help the patient reach the highest possible level of self-care.

6. **a.** The main purpose of the expected outcome statement is to describe the behavior that the patient is expected to achieve as a result of nursing interventions.

7. **b.** The components of the outcome statement are the patient's behavior, measurement criteria, conditions under which the behavior occurs, and a target date.

8. **b.** When developing nursing interventions, make your intervention statements specific to ensure continuity of care.

9. **c.** Unlike the standardized plan of care, which contains some preprinted information, the traditional plan of care is easy to individualize because it is written from scratch for each patient.

10. **d.** To develop an effective plan of care, establish realistic goals for each patient, individualize your approach to each patient's care, and avoid vague terminology.

Chapter 5: Implementation

1. **c.** Assessing a patient's financial and insurance status to determine if he meets eligibility requirements for receiving aid from government or community resources is an example of a socioeconomic intervention.

2. **b.** To improve time management skills, you should plan your shift activities in advance, learn to delegate, and care for yourself as well as your patients. However, you should not respond immediately to each patient request. In certain instances, responding to requests later is more efficient.

3. **c.** To act assertively and confidently without appearing aggressive, state what you mean, be mindful of your body language, and listen attentively. Do not answer praise with such phrases as "oh, it was nothing."

4. **d.** To give constructive criticism to a colleague, you should object only to actions that the other person can change, state your criticism as a suggestion or question, and voice your criticism as soon as possible. Do not begin with a mild apology.

5. **a.** Collaboration involves both parties modifying their behavior to solve a problem.

6. **c.** Promoting restricted accountability for nurses is not an effective strategy for enhancing nurse-doctor collaboration. Examples of effective strategies include establishing a joint practice committee, implementing integrated patient records, implementing primary nursing, and promoting continuing education for nurses.

7. **d.** When documenting the implementation phase, record nursing observations and interventions, the time that nursing interventions are performed, and patient responses to interventions.

8. **a.** A disadvantage of narrative progress notes is that they tend to be tedious and lengthy.

9. **b.** The main disadvantage of relying too heavily on flow sheets to document nursing interventions is that flow sheets may fragment the documentation record.

10. **c.** If you make the effort to research and find an appropriate support group for your patient and he refuses to attend, assess whether he can help himself without the support group or if he's just denying his problems and feelings.

Chapter 6: Evaluation

1. **d.** Evaluation, the last step in the nursing process, gives you the opportunity to make judgments about the quality and appropriateness of nursing care. This dynamic and ongoing process overlaps with other phases of nursing care.

2. **b.** The evaluation statement is important because it provides a means of substantiating the rationales for nursing care and justifying the use of nursing resources.

3. **c.** Objective evaluation is based on data you can observe and verify.

4. **a.** The most important determinant for reassessment is the patient's condition.

5. **c.** The purpose of a retrospective evaluation is to monitor the quality and efficiency of care.

6. **a.** A nursing diagnosis is resolved when the patient attains expected outcomes associated with the diagnosis.

7. **d.** When evaluating your patient, determine if the plan of care must be modified, if expected outcomes have been achieved and, if so, if they've been achieved by the target dates.

8. **d.** If the patient fails to achieve an expected outcome, assess factors that interfere with goal achievement, review implementation of the plan of care, and revise interventions, expected outcomes, or nursing diagnoses as needed.

9. **b.** Criteria used during evaluation are established during planning, the third step of the nursing process.

10. **c.** *Patient reports achieving pain relief 40 minutes after injection of meperidine hydrochloride 75 mg I.M.* is the best example of a clearly written evaluation statement.

Chapter 7: Discharge planning

1. **a.** In most cases, you would refer to hospital policy to determine who is responsible for discharge planning.

2. **b.** The major reason that discharge planning is becoming increasingly important is that the length of the average hospital stay is decreasing.

3. **c.** Begin evaluating a patient's need for postdischarge care during your initial assessment.

4. **e.** The implementation phase of discharge planning may involve referring your patient to a self-help group, providing written instructions for him to take home, teaching him and his family about home care procedures, and arranging for outside services.

5. **d.** Most patients receive the bulk of their postdischarge home care from family members and friends.

6. **b.** A psychiatrist is responsible for evaluating the patient's mental status to determine if competence is at issue.

7. **c.** If you wish to provide discharge instructions to an illiterate patient, use pictures to communicate your instructions.

8. **a.** If you feel that a patient about to leave the hospital is not adequately prepared for discharge, speak out to ensure the patient's safety and well-being.

9. **c.** If you're in the middle of performing a nursing procedure and the patient interrupts with a question about his care, provide an answer to the patient's question and follow up with more information later.

10. **b.** You perform an assessment of a patient's home environment because this environment can greatly affect his progress after discharge.

Chapter 8: Legal issues

1. **c.** The statement "once established and accepted by the nursing profession, standards are rarely changed" is false because as technology advances and nursing responsibilities expand, standards change as well. The other statements regarding nursing standards are true.

2. **d.** Under standards of the Joint Commission on Accreditation of Healthcare Organizations (JCAHO), you may use any of the formats listed (the problem-intervention-evaluation format, charting by exception, or narrative charting) to document your nursing care.

3. **c.** According to JCAHO recommendations, you should perform a weekly reassessment on a patient in long-term care.

4. **b.** If you're a defendant in a malpractice or negligence suit, your actions will be compared with those of a reasonably prudent nurse in a similar situation.

5. **d.** JCAHO standards require that each patient's care be based on identified nursing diagnoses or another documented format, such as a patient problem list.

6. **c.** If you make a mistake when writing in the clinical record, draw a single line through it, write "error" above or beside it, and sign and date your corrections.

7. **b.** According to standards of the American Nurses' Association (ANA), patient outcomes are derived from nursing diagnoses, not assessment data. Additionally, outcomes must be realistic in relation to the patient's capabilities, must be revised according to ongoing assessment findings, and should include a time estimate for attainment.

8. **c.** ANA standards carry significant weight in legal disputes because they represent a national consensus.

9. **b.** If a nurse realizes she forgot to document routine reassessment of a patient's vital signs, she should document the missing information and identify it as a late entry.

10. **a.** In cases of nursing negligence, national standards are being favored over local and state standards.

Chapter 9: Computers and the nursing process

1. **d.** Using a nursing information system can help you collect assessment data, develop a plan of care, and document progress notes.

2. **a.** To gain entry to a patient's computerized clinical record, you must enter a personal password called a signature code.

3. **c.** Current computer programs can provide a list of diagnoses along with associated assessment findings.

4. **b.** Computer terminals installed at the patient's bedside are known as point-of-care systems.

5. **c.** A data base is a collection of data in a form that facilitates retrieval and use of information.

6. **a.** A microprocessor is an integrated circuit containing the entire central processing unit of a computer.

7. **a.** A mainframe computer can provide access to numerous users simultaneously.

8. **b.** Computers improve the efficiency of the nursing process, allowing more time for direct patient care; help make patient information legible; and help link diverse sources of patient information, broadening the horizons of nursing research and allowing for nursing decisions to be made on a more scientific basis. Computers do not enhance the nurse-patient relationship by reinforcing the patient's belief that information will be kept confidential. Rather, they may threaten a patient's right to privacy if he feels that his history could be read by others without his knowledge or permission.

9. **c.** A nursing minimum data set (NMDS) would not facilitate instant consultation with nursing experts through an on-line bulletin board system. An NMDS would, however, be used to stimulate nursing research through links to data stored in nursing information systems, generate data about nursing care that can be used to influence health policy decisions, and validate the defining characteristics of nursing diagnoses more accurately.

10. **b.** The aim of those developing artificial intelligence is to create programs that simulate the human thinking process.

INDEX

i refers to illustration; t refers to table

B

Bathing, self-care deficit and, 251t
Belonging
  in Maslow's hierarchy of needs, 105i
  nursing diagnoses and, 106
Blood, assessment of, 32
Body image disturbance, 237t
Body language, use of, in communicating, 140
Body temperature alteration, high risk for, 237t
Bowel incontinence, 237t
Breast-feeding
  effective, 237t
  ineffective, 237t
  interrupted, 237t
Breasts, assessment of, 30
Breathing pattern, ineffective, 238t

C

Cardiac output, decreased, 239t
Cardiovascular system
  assessment of, 30
  physical examination of, 35
Caregiver role strain, 238t
  high risk for, 238t
Care plan. *See* Plan of care.

CBE. *See* Charting-by-exception format.
Charting-by-exception format, 154-157, 206
Charting format, selecting, 206
Choosing as human response pattern, 61t
Clarity, lack of, as documentation error, 212
Closed-ended documentation, 39, 41, 42
Clothes worn by patient, observing, 16
Code record as documentation tool, 151
Cognitive and perceptual pattern, 13, 15
Cognitive functions, observing, 16
Collaboration as conflict resolution strategy, 143
Collaborative interventions, 132
Collaborative practice, 146-147
  discharge planning and, 179-180
Colleagues, relationships with, 139-145
Comfort, promotion of, as nursing intervention, 133
Communicating as human response pattern, 60t
Communication
  impaired verbal, 238t
  observation of patient's ability for, 16
  patient interview and, 20-28

i refers to illustration; t refers to table

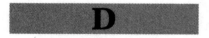

D

i refers to illustration; t refers to table

E

i refers to illustration; t refers to table

F

i refers to illustration; t refers to table

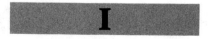

i refers to illustration; t refers to table

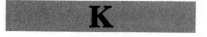

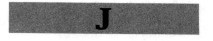

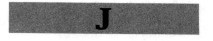

i refers to illustration; t refers to table

i refers to illustration; t refers to table

i refers to illustration; t refers to table

Q

i refers to illustration; t refers to table

i refers to illustration; t refers to table

T

i refers to illustration; t refers to table